Comments on **Gout – the 'at you**

from readers

'It is excellent as an information resource for patients and doctors.'

Dr Michael Snaith, Senior Lecturer in Rheumatology, University of Sheffield

'Here is a splendid book. All your questions answered!'

Ronald Simms, who has had gout for 36 years

GOUT

The 'at your fingertips' guide

Rodney Grahame CBE, MD, FRCP, FACP, FRSA
Consultant Rheumatologist, University College London Hospitals; Emeritus Professor of Clinical Rheumatology

H Anne Simmonds MSc PhD DipChemPath
Founder/Director Purine Research Unit, Guy's, Kings and St Thomas' Hospitals; Emeritus Senior Lecturer in Nucleotide Metabolism

Elizabeth Carrey BSc PhD
Purine Research Unit, Guy's Hospital, London; Former Lecturer in Biochemistry, University College, London

CLASS PUBLISHING • LONDON

Printing history
First published 2003
Reprinted 2003

The authors and publishers welcome feedback from the users of this book. Please contact the publishers.

Class Publishing, Barb House, Barb Mews, London W6 7PA, UK
Telephone: 020 7371 2119 [International +4420]
Fax: 020 7371 2878
Email: post@class.co.uk
Visit our website – www.class.co.uk

A CIP catalogue record for this book is available from the British Library.

ISBN 1 85959 067 5

Edited by Gillian Clarke

Cartoons by Jane Taylor

Line illustrations by David Woodroffe

Indexed by Valerie Elliston

Typeset by Martin Bristow

Printed and bound in Great Britain by Biddles Short Run Books, Kings Lynn

Contents

Acknowledgements

The authors thank the following for their invaluable assistance in compiling the answers and for providing a critical review of this book:

Dr David Bender, Department of Biochemistry, University College London

Andrew Brown and Val Brown for information on the wine trade

Professor Stewart Cameron CBE, Emeritus Professor of Renal Medicine, Guy's Hospital, London: our mentor for renal disease

Susan Davies, SRCh, for information on chiropody

Dr Patrick Dessein, Baragwanath Hospital, Soweto, South Africa

Dr John Duley and Dr Lynette Fairbanks, the Purine Research Unit, Guy's Hospital, London

Jill Ferrari, Lecturer, The London Foot Hospital

Judy Hilton, Appeals Officer, Department for Work and Pensions

Dr Graham Jackson, Consultant Cardiologist, Guy's and St Thomas' NHS Hospital Trust, London

Dr Arian Laurence, Department of Haematology, University College Hospital, London

Dr Gillian McCarthy, Chailey Heritage Clinical Services

Dr Dev Muckerjee, Department of Rheumatology, Royal Free Hospital, London

Dr Bill Robertson, Institute of Urology and Nephrology, University College Hospital, London

Dr Tom Scott, Emeritus Consultant Physician, Charing Cross Hospital, London: our mentor for gout

Dr Nelson Tang, Prince of Wales Hospital, Hong Kong

Professor Warren Turner, School of Health and Community Studies, University of Derby

Dr Margaret Ashwell, for permission to reproduce the Ashwell Shape Chart.

This book is based on the questions posed by people with gout and their families, and we thank especially Ronald Simms, David Jordan, and the numerous families we have met through our work and through PUMPA, the Purine Metabolic Patients' Association. We are especially indebted to PUMPA, which provides a patient support group for the different metabolic disorders under its umbrella, the most prevalent being gout in middle-aged men. We also acknowledge the gracious patronage of the late Princess Margaret, Countess of Snowdon, who encouraged the work of the Purine Research Unit for many years.

The authors are very grateful for the cheerful and efficient work of all involved in publishing this book, especially their editor, Gillian Clarke.

Introduction

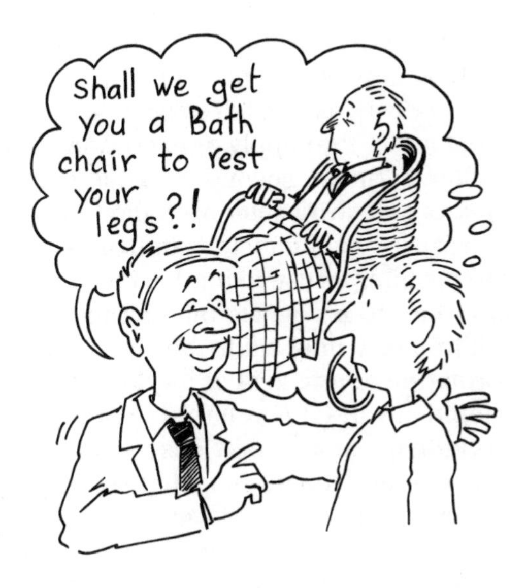

Some people may find that their friends greet a diagnosis of gout with great amusement: 'Lay off the port, dear boy!' they may say. 'Shall we get a Bath chair to rest your legs?' But the pain and swelling in joints (usually but not exclusively the big toe) are not amusing to the sufferer, especially when long periods of 'quiet' are followed by a sudden flare-up of painful and disabling symptoms.

What causes gout? Symptoms occur when high levels of uric acid or, rather, sodium urate accumulate in body fluids, forming crystals that are deposited in joints where they cause inflammation (gouty arthritis). Sodium urate may also be deposited in cartilage, in bones or under the skin.

Classic or 'primary' gout is almost exclusively a disease of adult men, because their kidneys excrete uric acid less well, and return more to the blood, than do the kidneys of women and children. However, gout is now being found in older women because many of the drugs used to treat high blood pressure (including diuretics – the 'water tablets') have the effect of diminishing the excretion of uric acid. Levels of uric acid rise in the blood, causing so-called 'secondary' gout. In the UK, gout affects 2.4 per 1,000 younger men, rising to about 30 per 1,000 at the age of 60. In the USA it has been suggested that gout is now the most common cause of inflammation in the joints of men over 40.

Secondary gout occurs as a result of several different illnesses or treatments that affect the supply or excretion of uric acid from the body. Another form of secondary gout ('saturnine' gout) prevalent in previous centuries is rare today, since the introduction of safety measures to eliminate lead from glass, water pipes and paint and to prohibit its use in food, wine or cosmetics.

It is also important to recognise that, although rare, gout can be found in children or young adults because of a faulty enzyme in either the formation of uric acid or its excretion. If this occurs, the person should always be referred to a specialist centre, because severe kidney damage may ensue. Gout in the young is always unusual, and must be investigated so that the cause, and other family members at risk of developing symptoms, can be identified. As in adults, the symptoms of gout can be managed or alleviated by drugs, and treatment will also help to prevent renal failure later on.

In this book we try to answer the important questions about the causes of gout and its management. Drugs are available to lower the levels of uric acid salts in the blood; to help to excrete uric acid from the kidneys; and to deal with the pain and inflammation. We also list foods to avoid, for those who wish to control gout symptoms through their diet.

1
What is gout?

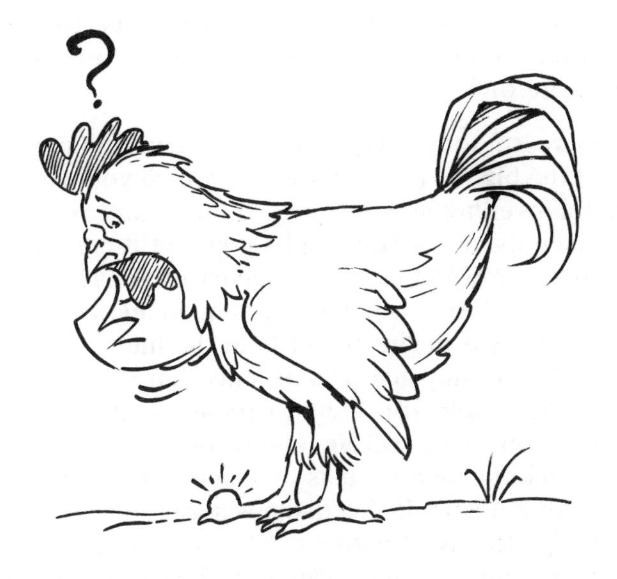

Gout can occur in anyone, irrespective of age or sex, when the level of uric acid or, rather, sodium urate in their blood rises above its 'solubility limit' so that crystals form in the body. Primary gout is typically seen in men aged 40–60, and the incidence is rising as our Western lifestyle leads to more obesity, heavier drinking and higher blood pressure. Gout symptoms are now found increasingly in women, too, as diuretic drugs are prescribed to more middle-aged and older women with high blood pressure. Gout symptoms may also be seen in people recovering from surgery or other stressful episodes, and gout is a possible complication of chemotherapy for cancer. Lead poisoning was a major cause of gout in the past, but it is much less common now.

This chapter addresses questions regarding the typical symptoms of gout and explains the reasons for the pain and swelling in the joints.

Diagnosing gout

My foot is so painful that I can't bear it to be touched. The doctor says that I've got podagra. What is this, and how long will it go on?

Podagra is a term for the gouty arthritis occurring in the joint at the base of the big toe (see Figure 1.1), which you will know is a very painful swelling accompanied by heat and redness in the skin. The pain usually settles on its own but it can take up to a week to do so, or even longer in some cases. This happens when it becomes 'migratory' – when it starts up in another (often adjacent) joint just as it begins to settle in the initial one. In severe cases your doctor may give you an injection of a corticosteroid (steroid) directly into the joint to reduce the swelling, which should give you relief within a day or two. This is usually reserved for a large joint such as the knee, where it is possible to combine taking a sample for diagnosis (see the next question) with a rapidly effective treatment. The pain of this procedure is minimised by using a local anaesthetic. You should also be taking

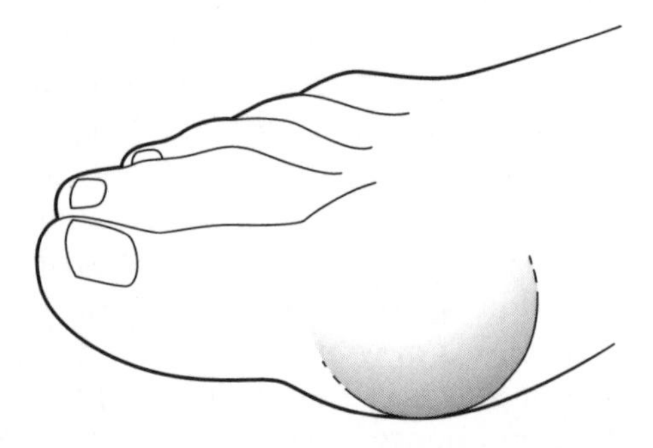

Figure 1.1 A swollen joint of the big (great) toe.

adequate anti-inflammatory drugs (see Chapter 3 for the best drugs for this purpose) or colchicine.

How can my doctor be sure that gout is what is the matter with me?

The typical signs of podagra, or gouty arthritis, are:

- sudden onset, often at night,
- excruciating pain that is worse on movement,
- hot, swollen, pink joint, often the big toe.

There are two steps to making the diagnosis of this condition. First, when you have an acute attack, a blood sample will be taken to measure the amount of urate in the plasma (your 'plasma urate level'). If the level has risen above 420 micromoles per litre (approximately equivalent to 7 milligrams per 100 millilitres – the highest amount of sodium urate that can dissolve in plasma), this can strongly suggest gout as the cause of the attack. Secondly, and especially if the attack does not have the typical hallmarks of podagra, a sample of fluid will be taken from the swollen joint and examined for crystals using a polarising microscope, which provides the only cast-iron diagnosis of gout. The fluid can be obtained using a syringe and needle under sterile conditions and is not as bad as it sounds! Most doctors use a local anaesthetic so that you feel only the first prick. A helpful spin-off is that removing most of the fluid instantly relieves the painful pressure within the joint.

What causes the swelling and pain in a gouty attack?

An accumulation of crystals of uric acid (or, more correctly, sodium urate) in the cavity of the joint attracts the attention of cells from the body's immune system. The immune cells are attracted into (infiltrate) the space around the joint, where they release chemicals called *cytokines*. In their fight against 'foreign bodies' (which includes micro-organisms, protein molecules and crystals), these cytokines cause swelling, heat and pain, which we know as inflammation. The skin over the inflamed joint is usually red and tender.

What is uric acid?

Uric acid is an end-product – the last chemical in a chain of steps that break down the purines from the genetic material (DNA and RNA) and the related chemical ATP which supplies energy within all our cells. These purine breakdown products are released into the blood from our cells as they die and are replaced, and purines are also released from food as it is digested. In the blood, 99 per cent of uric acid is in the form of the more soluble sodium urate. However, in urine, which has a wide range of acidity, the ratio of uric acid to urate varies, and it is almost entirely uric acid when the urine is very acidic. Thus, uric acid crystals and stones may also develop in the kidneys, leading to a decline in their efficiency.

Why do we have so much uric acid in our blood?

Uric acid is a chemical generated when purines – chemicals found in all our cells – are broken down during daily wear and tear. Most of our own purines are recycled for re-use by our cells. The problem is that our food contributes purines, which are broken down immediately in the gut membranes to create uric acid. Excess uric acid is then transported in the blood to the kidneys for the final steps of excretion, which involve the filtration and concentration of dissolved components of urine.

Thus primary gout arises when purine-rich food (e.g. offal, seafood) or drink (e.g. beer) is taken in a quantity that rapidly raises the level of uric acid in the blood to concentrations where no more can dissolve, so crystals form. Primary gout was very uncommon during the war years in 20th-century Europe, when food was scarce. This tells us two things: first, that the symptoms of primary gout may disappear when the diet is restricted; and second, that gout will become more common if a rich Western diet is adopted around the world. This has certainly been the case in Britain, where most people now eat a diet at least as rich and varied as that eaten by the overweight port-drinkers seen in the 18th-century cartoons. Similarly, people of Polynesian origin develop gout (and diabetes and high blood pressure) when they adopt Western-style eating habits. In some countries that have not adopted a 'rich' diet, for example China, primary gout is rare.

Is it possible for me to have gout even if my plasma urate levels are normal?

Yes. A possible explanation for this is that before and during an attack of acute gout there is a sudden transfer of sodium urate into the joint to form crystals, which temporarily depletes the amount of urate in the blood circulation. As a result the measurement of plasma urate falls into the 'normal' range. Not uncommonly, once the attack has passed, the level of plasma urate in the blood will rise again.

Can people have high levels of urate in their blood without developing gout symptoms?

Yes, it is possible to have a high level of urate in the blood (*hyperuricaemia*) but no gout symptoms. This can occur in people with renal failure – attributed to accumulation of as yet unknown factors that prevent the crystals from forming. Nevertheless, the higher the concentration of urate in the blood, the greater will be the chances of the crystals forming in the joint, resulting in gout. Paradoxically, in the presence of kidney damage, more uric acid is excreted directly via the gut, so the chances of an attack of acute gout are less.

Why does the body choose to convert excess uric acid into such unpleasant needle-like crystals?

Whereas common salt (sodium chloride) or sugar (sucrose) each form neat cubic crystals, sodium urate forms long, sharp crystals that give a distinctive pattern in polarised light under the microscope. Pain is not really caused by the shape of the crystals, but by the chemical attacks mounted by immune cells when they encounter the sodium urate crystals, causing heat and swelling in and around the joint.

My aunt has arthritis in her knees and her problems of pain and inflammation seem to be very like mine with gout. What is the difference between gout and arthritis?

Gout is an acute variety of arthritis. The word 'arthritis' simply means inflammation in a joint. Gout should be suspected when the first episode occurs 'overnight' and without any warning of prior stiffness. Typically, the first gouty attack involves the base of the big toe (great toe), but gouty arthritis may occur at other sites. Acute attacks are typically accompanied by a fever, flu-like symptoms or a stomach upset. The symptoms of gout usually subside completely between attacks in the early years. Later on, as the accumulation of urate in the tissues surrounding the joint continues relentlessly (in the absence of urate-lowering treatment) tophi (lumps) appear, and pain and swelling persist in between acute attacks. Uniquely, gout can be traced to the accumulation of a single waste product (uric acid) in the blood, so treatment to reduce this waste product is very effective in controlling the symptoms.

If I have gouty arthritis, does this mean I won't develop the other kinds of arthritis later?

The short answer is no! Sorry, but they have different causes, so there's no reason why you shouldn't get osteoarthritis or rheumatoid arthritis, for example, as well in the future. Damage to toe joints caused by gouty arthritis can in fact act as a focus for osteoarthritis in later life, so it is in your interests to keep this damage to a minimum. If, in addition to your regular drugs for gout, you maintain a healthy body weight, eat a healthy diet and exercise sensibly, you will be helping yourself to prevent many of the 'degenerative diseases' that we have seen become more common in older people.

I have had gout for several years and now I have found some fairly solid lumps on the top of my ear and on the back of my hand. Are these connected with gout?

A lump of urate salts is known as a *tophus*. As well as settling in the joints, these lumps *(tophi)* may be found on the edge of the outer ear, the back of the hand (see Figure 1.2), the elbow, the toes or the heel. Usually the lumps are seen in people who have chronic and long-standing gout, but occasionally a tophus under the skin is the first symptom of gout in someone with a related metabolic disorder (see Chapter 6, ***Gout in young people***) or in a middle-aged or older woman who has recently started taking diuretic drugs ('water tablets'). In some cases the tophus bursts through the skin, revealing a chalky deposit. The doctor may take a minute sample of the material with a syringe needle to confirm the identity of the deposit, as the distinctive crystals of uric acid will be visible under polarised light in the microscope.

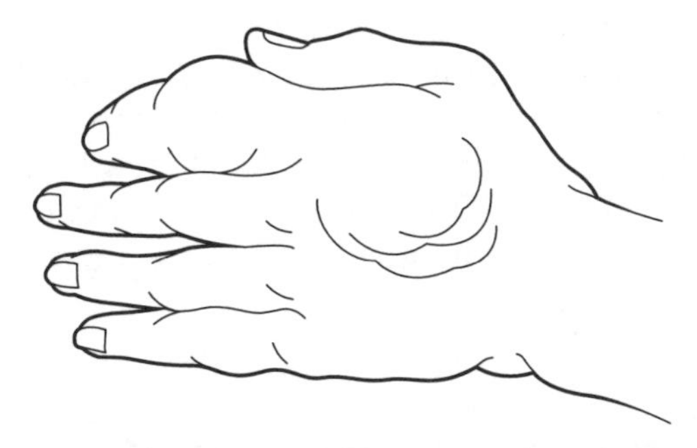

Figure 1.2 This person has developed a lump, or tophus, on the back of the hand and on the index finger.

I've had several gouty attacks that are preceded by 'leakage' from the edge of my ears. Is this uric acid?

Yes, the 'leaks' from your outer ear are composed of collections of excess sodium urate crystals or sodium urate in solution. In other people, such high concentrations of these chemicals will be deposited as a lump, called a tophus, in this position.

My uncle has been diagnosed with pseudo-gout – but his symptoms seem pretty real to me.

Some of the symptoms of pseudo-gout (also known as *chondrocalcinosis* or *pyrophosphate arthropathy*) are very similar to gout – the rapid onset of heat, pain and swelling in the affected joint, for example. However, this disorder occurs later in life, and usually affects a larger joint such as the knee. The attacks are similar to gout in that they arise from the formation of crystals in the joint. In pseudo-gout, however, the crystals are the chalk-like calcium pyrophosphate dihydrate, occasionally forming when there is too much calcium in the blood (*hypercalcaemia*) – such as occurs when the parathyroid gland is working overtime (*hyperparathyroidism*) or when the person consumes too much vitamin D. It may also occur with the disease known as *haemochromatosis*, in which too much iron is deposited in the liver and other organs. There is no link with purine-rich food or with excretion through the kidneys.

Some aspects of the treatment of pseudo-gout are the same as for gout – anti-inflammatory drugs, removing fluid (aspiration) from the affected joint and injection of corticosteroid. Attacks subside within a few days. The doctor may remove some fluid to confirm the diagnosis, as the crystals of calcium pyrophosphate dihydrate can easily be distinguished from sodium urate under the polarising microscope.

What brings on an attack of gout?

I had a gout attack following severe gut pain. Was the problem in my gut a cause or an effect of high levels of uric acid?

Gout may be triggered by any acute illness, and whatever caused the pain in your gut may also be acting as such a trigger. If your pain was due to food poisoning, that or the resulting dehydration could be the explanation. Although some uric acid is disposed of via the intestine (in faeces – your bowel movements), there is nothing to suggest that it can cause pain in the gut.

I don't drink heavily or over-eat, so I don't understand why I have had an attack of gout.

Purine-rich food and beer, especially real ale, can precipitate a gouty attack but may not be the only cause. Dehydration, heavy exercise, stress and several medicines can trigger these effects. If you are a young man in good health, it is possible that you have a mild form of a metabolic disorder (see Chapter 6, ***Gout in young people***) causing a naturally high level of uric acid in your blood, and an extra factor triggered your first gouty attack. Try to restrict the purine-containing foods in your diet (see Chapter 5, ***Food and drink***), and if your plasma urate level does not drop, ask your GP to refer you to a rheumatology or renal (kidney) unit that specialises in purine disorders. You can find some further information from the organisations listed in Appendix 1 (***Useful addresses***) of this book, including the PUMPA website.

Why is an attack of gouty arthritis so sudden, if all that stuff has been accumulating in the blood for years?

Hyperuricaemia (high levels of urate in the blood) can be present for many years without causing any symptoms. A number of different events or situations may then trigger an attack of gout. These include an injury, a surgical operation, or a binge of eating or drinking. Some people are very sensitive to some specific foods, and have wisely chosen to avoid them (for more about food and drink, see Chapter 5).

Why do the painful attacks of gouty arthritis come and go?

Sodium urate crystals can re-dissolve if or when their concentration in the plasma falls, and the excess is excreted through the kidneys. However, the concentration may rise again and more sodium urate may be deposited, causing a repeat of the symptoms.

Different forms of gout

Why is gout so much more common in men than in women?

Primary gout is more common in men because of a change at puberty, which results in the kidneys pulling more uric acid back into the blood. Urate levels in the blood rise at puberty in both sexes but to a considerably higher level in men. However, there are rare inherited conditions, where over-production of purines in the body leads to primary gout in both sexes in children and young people; these are described in Chapter 6 (***Gout in young people***).

If there is 'primary' gout, I expect there must be 'secondary' gout. What is that?

Secondary gout can be seen in people of either sex and at any age. It has the same symptoms, arising from *hyperuricaemia*, or high levels of urate in the blood, but in this case the gout has other causes:

- another disorder, such as glycogen storage disease, methyl malonic aciduria, or fructose intolerance,
- prescribed drugs such as diuretics (see Chapter 4, ***Drugs to lower the level of urate in the blood***), and pyrazinamide used for tuberculosis, which interfere with the excretion of uric acid from the kidneys,
- the destruction of cells through chemotherapy or physical damage,
- poisoning by lead (saturnine gout).

Surely lead poisoning is no longer a hazard? I remember when my parents had to have all the lead plumbing stripped out of their old house, and that was many years ago.

Lead pipes used for water coming into the house, or lead in the storage tanks, should have been eliminated from all old houses as their systems were upgraded. The pipes and tanks caused a danger from lead salts dissolved in the drinking water. The downfall of the Roman Empire was partly blamed on lead poisoning, which can result in kidney damage, mental illness and, of course, gout.

Lead paint can still be found under more recent layers, or in old buildings that have not been repainted for 30 years or so. Stripping the paint down to the bare wood will cause dangerous dust to be released, so masks should be worn and the debris should be disposed of as toxic waste. Be careful that children do not nibble on old painted toys or furniture, or on old paint that may flake off old doors.

My father and grandfather had gout, but I think that my attacks started at an earlier age than my father's disease. If it runs in the family, are my younger brother and his son at risk?

Many men with primary gout have a relative with the same condition – but it is not known to what extent genetic or lifestyle factors cause the link in any one person. Usually, urate levels have been high for many years before the capacity of their kidneys is exceeded and urate crystals begin to be deposited. You are probably better fed and less active than your grandfather and father were, so perhaps you have a higher plasma urate level earlier in life. Your brother and his son may not suffer gouty attacks if their other risk factors (obesity, high intake of purine, high blood pressure) are low.

Note that gout will 'run in the family' of people with the rare disorders described in Chapter 6 (***Gout in young people***). It would be wise to ensure that these metabolic causes have been ruled out, especially if your first gouty attack occurred when you were in your teens or twenties, and if you are worried about the future health of the next generation.

My daughter, in her twenties, has had an attack of gouty arthritis. I thought gout affected only middle-aged men?

Women before the menopause are usually protected from gout because the normal levels of the female sex hormone oestrogen help to promote the excretion of uric acid from the kidneys. After the menopause, levels of oestrogen fall unless hormone replacement therapy (HRT) is undertaken, and women may have their first attack of gout in late middle age (older than first attacks in men). Gout in a young woman is therefore unexpected, and your daughter should see her doctor and ask to be investigated for a metabolic disorder (see Chapter 6, ***Gout in young people***) rather than assuming that it is simply a defect in the excretion of uric acid.

My 75-year-old aunt has lumps on her ears and one hand, which came on after starting drugs for high blood pressure. This has been diagnosed as gout, so will she have attacks of gouty arthritis as well?

Gout is becoming much more common in middle-aged and older women, especially those who are prescribed diuretic drugs ('water tablets'). As mentioned earlier, women are better excretors of uric acid than men, but some blood pressure drugs, especially diuretics, decrease the body's ability to excrete uric acid. Attacks of acute gouty arthritis are not commonly seen in older women. The disease in this situation is usually called *tophaceous gout* (the lumps are called tophi; one lump is a tophus). Some tophi may be large and unsightly lumps on the back of the hands; others may lurk in the skeleton, causing damage that will be evident on x-ray pictures.

Can gout arise suddenly as a result of a serious illness?

Yes, this can happen but it is uncommon. Uric acid is formed from purines released when cells die at the end of their normal life span and it passes into the blood system. Thus, the wasting that may occur after a serious accident or major operation or, more important, cancer and cancer therapy can lead to hyperuricaemia, gout and possibly kidney failure. In cancer itself, both the growth and the death of cells occur much faster than usual. Some cancers, for example one that has spread to bone from another site, destroy nearby cells while they themselves are in the process of multiplying. Thus the rate of urate production rapidly exceeds the capacity of the kidneys to excrete it, which can lead to hyperuricaemia and gout. This is a form of secondary gout – the gout is a consequence of another disease.

Cancer treatment usually involves chemotherapy (with drugs) or radiotherapy (with x-rays). As a result, large numbers of tumour cells are killed quickly, with the release of vast amounts of purines. There may be a rapid rise of uric acid levels in blood and urine, and secondary gout may follow, as may acute kidney damage caused by uric acid crystals blocking the collecting ducts in the kidneys (the kidney tubules). As in any situation with an abnormally high level of uric acid (hyperuricaemia), tophi may also appear in the ears, under the skin and around the joints in such people. About 5 per cent of gout patients seen by hospital rheumatologists have high concentrations of uric acid derived from cells being destroyed by chemotherapy. To reduce this risk, many cancer specialists recommend the use of allopurinol (see Chapter 4, ***Drugs to lower the level of urate in the blood***) at the same time as cancer therapy. The dose must be carefully judged in these cases and in the people described in Chapter 6 (***Gout in young people***), because xanthine (the side-product from the use of allopurinol) may also form stones and could lead to acute kidney (renal) failure. Some cancer specialists inject a preparation of an enzyme – uricase – which will remove uric acid from the blood system of people having therapy. This treatment is described in more detail in Chapter 7 (***Research and the future***).

My daughter is studying to be a vet, and she says that some animals can get gout. Is she having me on?

No, she's right. Birds excrete very concentrated uric acid – the white part of their droppings. An inbred strain of chicken with a deficiency in urate excretion gets really unsightly lumps on its legs and feet as a result of uric acid deposits. They are disabled – and not as cute as the cartoon chickens in this book! Likewise, uric acid is the end-product of nitrogen metabolism in snakes and lizards, and you can imagine the problems encountered by gouty snakes! Palaeontologists have evidence – presumably from fossil bones – that dinosaurs suffered from gout.

Curiously, humans, higher apes and some varieties of dogs, such as the Dalmatian, are the only mammals to have significant amounts of uric acid in their blood. Dalmatians usually excrete the uric acid very efficiently, but they are prone to uric acid stones in the kidneys. The dogs can be treated by restricting the purines in their diet, by giving allopurinol to slow the conversion to uric acid and by making the urine less acidic to keep up the solubility of the uric acid – much like humans, in fact. Interestingly, excreting uric acid in place of a more soluble (and smelly) chemical makes Dalmatians good hunting dogs – other species cannot detect them by their odour!

Gout and the kidneys

The doctors say that my kidney stones are probably linked to my gout. What is the connection?

Because it is not very soluble, uric acid is also deposited as 'stones' or an accumulation of crystals in the kidneys of some people with gout, especially if their urine is very acid – as it often is in the gouty. If the stones remain in the kidneys, they may increase the risk of infection in a kidney or other parts of the urinary tract. If a stone passes along the ureter (the tube from the kidney to the bladder) but is too big to travel with the urine, it may cause severe pain and obstruct the flow of urine, leading to kidney damage caused by the rising pressure (called back-pressure) in the collecting system.

I developed diabetes a few years ago, and my GP suspects that my kidneys may have become damaged. Will this lead to gout?

Arterial disease is quite commonly a result of Type 2 (non-insulin-dependent) diabetes that develops in adults, especially those who are overweight and have high blood pressure. This often runs in families. If the circulation of your kidneys is affected, it may reduce the efficiency of their filtration process. This means that if you are at risk – through a high-purine diet or an increased production of uric acid – you might have an attack of gout. You should follow the advice on diet and exercise you are given to deal with the diabetes, and also try to maintain a low intake of purines (see Chapter 5, ***Food and drink***). Ask your doctor to check the levels of urate in your plasma.

Have my kidneys suffered permanent damage as a result of gout? Or will they improve if I use the drugs and follow the diet that my doctor suggests?

A mild degree of kidney damage can occur in people with gout but this does not necessarily imply that their kidneys are badly affected or that it will progress to kidney failure. Admittedly, there are some people who have developed a kidney disease resulting in hyperuricaemia and secondary gout, but these are different from people with ordinary gout, who may have only a mild degree of kidney damage.

Uric acid crystals may be deposited in the kidneys of some people who have a particularly pronounced type of hyper-uricaemia, arising from inherited conditions linked to a gene on the X chromosome. The first symptoms from these conditions generally appear in childhood (see under 'Incidence and diagnosis', in Chapter 6, ***Gout in young people***).

2
Living with gout

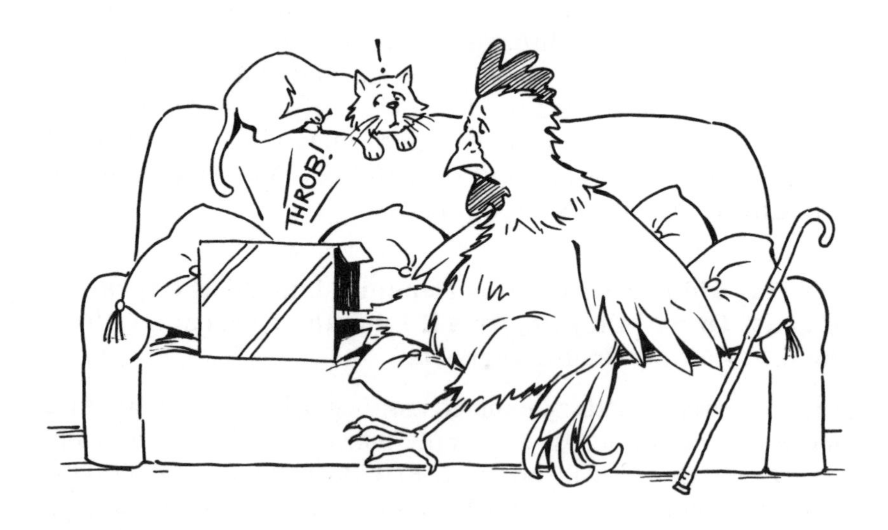

Gout, if untreated, used to develop into *chronic tophaceous gout*, a very painful condition often associated with severe damage to the joints similar to that seen in rheumatoid arthritis. With modern treatment, however, it is possible to lead a near-normal life with gout.

The acute attack

My first attack of gouty arthritis was very painful so I phoned my GP, who luckily was able to visit me at home within a few hours. Should I have got someone to drive me to the Emergency department of the hospital (25 miles away)?

It's essential to get rapid treatment when joints suddenly become hot and painful, with red–blue coloration and swelling. It may be gout – but it needs to be distinguished from septic (infectious) arthritis because the treatment will be quite different. So if your GP cannot see you quickly, it would not be unreasonable to go to your nearest hospital Accident & Emergency department.

Are there any symptoms I ought to look out for as an early warning of acute attacks?

Many people report a fever and general 'unwell' feeling when a gouty attack is imminent. This is probably the effect of chemical substances released in the blood as a result of the body's immune response. Some people have a gouty attack shortly after a stomach upset; or they notice that their urine is very yellow, which could be a sign of dehydration, so always drink plenty of water, especially if you have had alcoholic drinks.

What brings on an acute attack of gouty arthritis? I seem to get more attacks during the winter.

Your getting more attacks in winter could be explained on the basis of 'stress' from bacterial or viral infection, the tendency to eat more (especially 'comfort' foods) in winter, or drinking more beer and spirits in the Christmas and New Year season. However, in summer there is more likelihood of getting dehydrated from hot weather or intensive exercise, which can also provoke an acute gouty attack.

Now that I have got over my first couple of attacks of gout I seem to be OK on the drugs they gave me at the hospital. Do I call my GP if I have another attack, or should I ask to be referred to the hospital again?

When all goes to plan, the treatment of gout can be very satisfactory. Most GPs are familiar with this disease and its treatment, so in most cases it is not necessary to go to hospital for gout treatment on a regular basis. Your GP can provide all the care and prescribe all the drugs you need to keep your condition under control. Most people with gout fare very well in this way.

However, not everyone with gout responds in the standard way, and some may continue to suffer attacks of gout in spite of being prescribed the correct drugs. When a GP recommends further help, the appropriate hospital specialist for this purpose is a consultant rheumatologist.

Dealing with work and gout

I find it very frustrating that my colleagues can't take my gout seriously. I had a bad gouty attack the day after the office Christmas party and I had to take a week off work. Of course, this gave the impression that I was lying low with a bad hangover, and I worry that it will count against me when bonuses and promotion are discussed with my boss.

Gout has been a feature of cartoons and sketches, with the stereotype of the gluttonous drunkard, perhaps in a Bath chair, for at least 200 years, and is still not regarded as 'serious' by non-sufferers. You should discuss the subject with your line manager or other senior colleagues when you are between attacks. Point out that your mental capacity is still intact during an acute gouty attack, and that once the pain is under control you will be able to use the telephone and computer to keep in touch with the office. At next year's party, be careful to avoid purine-rich foods, using the advice in Chapter 5 (***Food and drink***), and restrict your alcohol intake to within healthy limits. Make sure that the office gossip sees that you are drinking several glasses of mineral water!

My job as a sales rep involves a lot of driving and then walking around to get to offices. Obviously I work from home on days when I have had a gouty attack, and my boss is happy with this. However, I wonder if the regular driving is having any effect on my feet that might make them more vulnerable to podagra.

Presumably you have been supplied with an 'automatic' so that you don't have to use your foot to change gear. If you are using a manual ('shift') car, ask to have it changed to an automatic.

In fact, it's more likely that sitting in the car is depriving you of exercise. You are also probably eating irregular meals, perhaps burgers or the 'wrong' kind of food (see Chapter 5, ***Food and drink***), and you may find it difficult to drink enough fluid during your working day. Be sure to drink enough water; and don't unwind by drinking alcohol in the evening. Take some fruit with you as a snack while on the road, and stop the car from time to time to stretch your legs or take a stroll.

My brother gets very depressed when his podagra flares up. Can he take anything for the depression?

Some people feel 'out of sorts' in a variety of ways just before an attack of gout. Sometimes this feels like depression. This is an early warning of an attack and should allow him to start his anti-inflammatory drugs before the attack gets really established and to avoid making things worse by drinking alcohol or taking purine-rich foods. It does not represent a form of depressive illness and therefore should not need treatment with antidepressant drugs.

If he is already depressed for other reasons, he may be taking antidepressant drugs for a few months. But by and large they do not interfere with any of the drugs used in the treatment of gout. The widely available *Hypericum* (St John's wort) preparations are herbal remedies that, though not licensed as medicines, have a proven effect on mild depression. Commercial preparations of St John's wort may have different levels of the active ingredient and can interfere with other medicines or can stop them working properly. It is probably best if your brother does not use St John's wort if he is taking any other drug prescribed by his doctor, or at least discusses it with his doctor first.

Deposits of sodium urate in the joints

I'm fascinated – in a gruesome way – with the idea of urate salts being quietly deposited in my joints. Will x-rays help to show up any less obvious urate deposits?

X-rays are used principally to assess the possible damage to the joints in long-term (chronic) gout. In the early stages of gout, the joints look normal on an x-ray. Urate deposits are not opaque to x-rays (radio-opaque), unlike calcium pyrophosphate in pseudo-gout, which is very radio-opaque. Urate deposits may acquire a patchy coating of calcium salts, and then they may show up on x-rays.

A diagnosis of *tophaceous gout* implies a more severe disease than non-tophaceous gout. Where no tophi are seen externally on the ears, elbows or around the joints, an x-ray can show them up in the bones adjacent to an affected joint. Sometimes a tophus may be formed in the joints of the hands or between vertebrae, where it may affect a nerve without causing an acute arthritis and without being visible externally. The damage to or erosion of the bone caused by such a tophus would show up on x-rays.

Why does gout affect some joints, especially the big toe, and not others?

In areas far from the heart where the blood is passing in tiny blood vessels (capillaries), blood flow is restricted and the temperature is slightly lower: these conditions encourage the sodium urate to be deposited as crystals. This is why the joints in the extremities (feet and, sometimes, hands) are the most common places for deposits. In half of all first attacks, only one joint is affected; this is referred to as *monoarticular gout*. If several joints are affected, it will be referred to as *polyarticular gout*.

Should I strap up my painful toe joint and just try to get on with things, or should I rest my foot?

When your foot is really agonisingly painful, you won't want to walk around and should definitely rest it. You can have a warm bath or use a warm pack on the foot – but make sure it is not so hot that you scald the skin and underlying tissue. Podiatrists (foot specialists, who might also be called chiropodists) don't encourage the use of cold packs for gouty inflammation, because they may tend to encourage the urate crystals to form. However, cold packs are effective at reducing the pain and you may find it easier to lay your hands on a bag of frozen peas than a hot water bottle. Gradually you will be able to put weight on your foot and to walk around gingerly.

If you decide to use a walking stick, be sure that it is the correct length to be used without bending your arm or twisting your body. The top of the stick should be on a level with your wrist when your arm is hanging straight down. Best support is given by using the stick on the same side as your *unaffected* foot; then the stick can take your weight, like an extra leg, instead of the gouty foot.

Once the pain has subsided enough, what is the best way for me to get around?

As an acute attack draws to a close, you will need to wear soft and comfortable shoes to accommodate swollen joints, and they should be easy to get into – soft slip-ons, or trainer-style with a Velcro or buckle closure rather than lace-ups – or, if worse comes to worst, bedroom slippers! Look for shoes with a rigid sole, or use a specially made insole to help to absorb the shock of contact with the ground and to restrict bending of your toe. For regular temporary swelling or for more permanent deformity causing pain or difficulty in walking, a podiatrist (see the previous answer) can help by relieving pressure with padding, reducing the size of corns, advising on footwear or providing supports for inserting into your shoes. Shoes can be made wider, or a 'balloon patch' can be inserted into your shoe's upper near to a very swollen or deformed joint, to relieve the pressure. Although specially made shoes can be very costly, 'semi-orthopaedic' shoes can be obtained at a more reasonable price and with a more acceptable appearance.

If you have to wear boots with steel toecaps at work, you may find that they cannot accommodate more than a small amount of swelling or deformity. Ask your podiatrist for advice on getting a larger pair or perhaps on adjusting the reinforcement (a steel balloon patch?).

How can I find a podiatrist who specialises in gouty feet?

In the past, the NHS podiatry service was available only to people of pensionable age or under 16, but nowadays anyone who needs it should get access to the service. However, in practice, each area in the UK will have slightly different patterns of service. Areas that receive good funding will have a full range of podiatry services – children, sports injuries, biomechanics (as in flat feet or other foot deformities), nail surgery, foot surgery, orthotics (provision of arch supports) – as well as the rheumatology, diabetes and geriatric services.

Your area's NHS podiatry service will usually be found at the local/principal hospital and will be called the Chiropody or Podiatry Department or the Foot Health Department (in an effort to avoid confusion over the names Chiropody and Podiatry!). Your GP should also know the address, and in fact some GPs now provide a service for their patients in their own centre.

It is important to know that all state-registered podiatrists will have the letters 'SRCh' (for State Registered Chiropodist). You should check this if you decide on private treatment, as the profession is also open to practitioners without the same level of training.

Even if I can get rid of the excess uric acid from my joints, will my feet be permanently deformed?

That depends on how badly deformed they were when you started treatment. Deposits of urate crystals in the joints will cause pain and swelling but the inflammation should always 'resolve' itself completely if the urate is removed from circulation. Feet sometimes deform if urate is deposited in clumps in the tissues of the foot outside the joint, distorting the shape of the foot. If tophi form within the bones of the feet, considerable ('gross') deformity can be caused. This can result in more severe problems and even make it very difficult to walk. Sometimes tophi can burst through the skin of the foot and, because the uric acid impedes healing, the open sore can become infected. If this happens to you, you should see your podiatrist or GP as quickly as possible!

Other things being equal, as urate-lowering treatment progresses, larger tophi diminish in size and smaller tophi may disappear altogether. Without urate-lowering treatment (see Chapter 4, ***Drugs to lower the level of urate in the blood***) permanent stress on the joints can result in fused joints or secondary osteoarthritis in the foot.

My podagra attacks seem to occur early in the morning when I am in bed. My feet often feel cold at night, as I have poor circulation. Should I wear socks in bed and generally try to keep my feet warm?

You mention that your feet feel cold at night due to poor circulation. This could also be caused by narrowing of the arteries, in turn linked to smoking or diabetes, so you may consider cutting down on cigarettes and watching your diet if these apply to you. Wearing bed socks may be more comfortable for your feet, and the extra warmth may prevent the urate from forming crystals in the toe joints. If you don't already use a duvet, you may find that a good one keeps you warmer than sheets and blankets, and there will be less weight on your feet to restrict the flow of blood.

Continuing healthcare

How did my GP decide which drugs to put me on when I had my first attack? Will they prevent attacks in the future?

Once a first attack has settled and the affected joint has returned to normal, the question arises as to whether it is advisable to take active steps to prevent future attacks. If it is decided to take this route, there are two possibilities. The first is by taking a drug such as *colchicine*, or a non-steroidal anti-inflammatory drug (*NSAID*; e.g. ibuprofen), on a low-dose long-term basis, to treat the symptoms of gouty arthritis (see Chapter 3, ***Drugs to combat pain and inflammation***). Many people get along very well with this kind of treatment and some modifications to their diet and exercise.

The more thorough way to prevent future attacks is to lower the concentration of uric acid in the blood system (see Chapter 4, ***Drugs to lower the level of urate in the blood***). There are two types of drug that can achieve this:

- **uricosuric drugs**, which increase the excretion of urate by the kidneys, thus lowering the concentration in the blood, and
- **xanthine oxidase inhibitors**, usually *allopurinol*, which reduce the formation (and, hence, the build-up) of urate in blood and urine.

Reducing the plasma urate levels to normal by either means reduces the risk and incidence of further attacks. Whether the drug treatment does abolish gouty attacks altogether depends partly on the doctor getting the dose right and partly on you taking the tablets regularly and diligently according to the doctor's instructions. Some people think they are cured when the attack subsides with treatment, and they may be tempted to stop taking allopurinol if a long time elapses with no sign of another attack. This is not a good idea, though. If allopurinol is prescribed for you, you must take it regularly.

I had a series of gouty attacks a couple of years ago. Nothing has happened since. Am I likely to have another attack if I stop taking the drugs my doctor prescribed?

There is a risk that, if you stop taking the drugs, your plasma urate level will rise and the gouty attacks may recur. It might be a risk you are prepared to take in order to avoid having to take drugs for the rest of your life, which, in itself, is quite a major undertaking! However, if in the meantime you have changed your lifestyle by losing weight, stopping drinking and cutting down on purine-rich food, it could be worth a try, but ask your doctor before stopping (or cutting down on) your prescribed drugs. Some people – about 10 per cent – only ever have one gouty attack, and in their case allopurinol has no advantage over these lifestyle changes. Others may have repeated attacks, which become more frequent and longer-lasting as time goes by, even with continuing drug treatment.

Will the gout get worse as I get older?

Not necessarily. Provided that your plasma urate level is well controlled (and this means taking your tablets regularly), you should become free of attacks within 6–12 months of commencing urate-lowering drugs. Tophi will gradually begin to get smaller and your tendency to produce uric acid kidney stones will also diminish. Well-controlled gout is a state that should last for the rest of your life. There is a tendency in old age for the kidneys to lose some of their ability to excrete uric acid and other waste products. This should not affect the control of gout as described above, unless other factors arise such as your kidneys being damaged by some other disease or if you start to take drugs (e.g. diuretics or NSAIDs) that may alter the way the kidneys handle urate.

My doctor has been monitoring my blood pressure while he is treating me for gout but I don't understand why. What is the connection?

It has been known for more than half a century that high blood pressure and hyperuricaemia are often found in the same person. They both occur in families, meaning that both have a hereditary tendency. Doctors know that these two conditions commonly occur together in the same individual, and finding one should raise a suspicion of the other. Drugs that treat one do not help the other; on the other hand, diuretics given for high blood pressure may induce an acute gout attack. Raised blood pressure is a potentially serious condition that, if untreated, may lead to stroke or coronary heart disease, both of which can be prevented by effective and timely drug treatment and a modified lifestyle. Many aspects of the lifestyle adopted to control blood pressure will also help to control gout symptoms. That is why your doctor is keeping an eye on your blood pressure when you consult him over your gout.

I've been having problems getting an erection. Are there any known connections between gout or gout medication and impotence?

Gout as such does not cause impotence (erectile dysfunction, or ED) but some of the diseases that often accompany gout may result in erectile dysfunction. In this context diabetes and hypertension (high blood pressure) are more likely to be responsible. We know that a high level of uric acid is a risk factor for coronary disease, and so a gouty man may have ED, which could be an early indication of coronary heart disease or diabetes. This possibility should be discussed with your GP, who may already have been investigating your blood pressure (see the previous question).

Regarding drugs used in the treatment of gout, there have been no reports of ED connected with allopurinol, colchicine or probenecid. On the other hand, anti-inflammatory drugs inhibit processes involved in the control of erection of the human penis, and there have been reports of dysfunction connected with prescription of indometacin or naproxen. Your GP should be able to prescribe a different pain-killer for your gouty attacks.

Advice on treatment of ED may be obtained locally from Genito-Urinary Medicine clinics, or you can look at the website at www.impotence.org.uk. The first clinic in the UK dedicated to cardiovascular health for men and also catering for ED problems is at Guy's Hospital, London, directed by Dr Graham Jackson, author of *Heart Health – the 'at your fingertips' guide*, in this series.

Recuperation and exercise

The manager of my local health food shop recommends glucosamine sulphate as a help for pain and immobility in osteoarthritis. Do you think it would help the same symptoms in my gout?

Glucosamine sulphate is a natural component of the cartilage in our joints, helping the surfaces of the bones to move smoothly against each other. In your case, if the sodium urate crystals have damaged the surfaces of your joints, some damage may remain even if the crystals have been cleared, and the joints may feel 'stiff'. Many doctors are sceptical about this product but you have probably seen enthusiastic testimonials from people who feel that their arthritis has been eased. There is no scientific evidence that taking glucosamine sulphate by mouth helps gout, or any other form of arthritis for that matter. Except that it can affect diabetes, as far as we know it seems to be harmless.

When my husband is laid up with his gout, he has to cancel his regular squash games, and he worries that his general fitness will be harmed. Can he do any exercises that will help?

He can continue to exercise other parts of his body, for example using hand weights. Obviously he can't do press-ups but he could do pull-ups. For aerobic exercise, he may find that swimming is better than squash anyway, because it exercises the whole body without putting weight or stress on his feet. He should certainly keep up exercise in the periods between acute attacks, because this helps to keep his weight down.

Should I take up some walking or running exercise in between attacks to help to get the crystals moving instead of being deposited in my toe joints?

Walking is recommended, but running involves much more pressure on the joints (especially those of the big toe) and could spell trouble – it may set off an attack of podagra. Cycling is another efficient way of getting from A to B, and it does not entail the use of the big toe joint, which is vulnerable in people with gout. If traffic in your area makes it dangerous to cycle, you might like to invest in an exercise bike; although there won't be any scenery to admire, you can always read a book as you cycle!

Are there any gadgets or pieces of equipment that can help when my joints are really painful? I put my foot up on the sofa and it seems to act as a magnet for the cat and small children – agony, as you can imagine.

You may well feel that any touch, even from the lightest bedclothes, is too much to bear. The cheapest gadget might be a cardboard box – try a sturdy box that a small electrical appliance was packed in – as long as you have space to put your foot inside and to move it slightly as you rest or sleep. When you sit with your foot up on the sofa, place the box over your foot, making sure that it covers your foot completely. Don't make the box look inviting to your cat, and keep it out of the way when not in use.

Adjustable beds and chairs are available, whose angle can be altered to give you a change of position. Such a chair can cost several hundred pounds, so ask your local social services department or Department for Work and Pensions (formerly the Benefits Agency) if you can get any help with their purchase. If you are receiving Income Support, the DWP may be able to give you help from the Social Fund. Many gadgets are available –

some by mail order – for reaching out when you are confined to bed or the sofa, and you may find some useful. You can also use the remote control for the TV, video or radio. Telephone your nearest Disabled Living Centre (look in your phone book), and make an appointment to visit and discuss any help or aids you need. The organisation REMAP makes or adapts aids, when not commercially available, for people with disabilities (contact details in Appendix 1, ***Useful addresses***).

We are looking forward to a holiday in the sun but the attacks are so unpredictable. Will the drugs help us plan for next summer?

Regular use of urate-lowering drugs should keep things on an even keel if you don't change your drugs, diet or exercise regimen drastically while you are away! Eat carefully, drink lots of water to avoid becoming dehydrated, and watch out for gastric upsets causing diarrhoea and/or vomiting (you may encounter a different group of bugs from those at home). Keep the information leaflet from your regular drugs and strong pain-killers with you in case of emergency. Some antibiotics are available without a prescription in parts of Europe, and because some (e.g. ampicillin) may interfere with the action of urate-lowering drugs, you should make sure that the pharmacist is aware of your regular medication.

The worst problem would be to have an acute gouty attack just before or during a journey. If you alert the airline in advance they can provide a wheelchair in the airport. They may provide you with extra leg-room if you have a gouty attack during the flight, provided there is space on the aircraft.

Asking for financial help

Am I eligible for free NHS prescriptions or a reduced prescription charge?

As with all NHS prescriptions, you don't have to pay the

prescription charge if you are:

- under the age of 16,
- aged 16, 17 or 18 and in full-time education,
- aged 60 or over,
- pregnant,
- receiving any of certain state benefits (e.g. Income Support).

Check the information on the back of the prescription form or ask the pharmacist for the current rules.

If you are required to pay the prescription charge, this can be a significant sum over the years, so it is worth thinking about ways of saving money. First, you can ask to have an annual 'season ticket' for the charges, which will be worthwhile if you receive more than 15 prescriptions in a year (that is, more than 15 separate items). Season tickets lasting four months are also available. At the time of writing the annual charge is £89, or £32.40 for four months. Secondly, you could ask your doctor if a private prescription (where you pay the actual price of the drugs) would be cheaper than the NHS prescription charge. This could be especially useful if you are getting prescriptions every month for a fairly cheap drug; if you then find that a three-month supply costs more than the NHS charge, you could ask your doctor to give you prescriptions for three months' worth of drugs and go back to NHS prescriptions.

When I have a gouty attack, I really cannot get about. Would I be eligible for the Disability Living Allowance benefit?

In the UK, Disability Living Allowance (DLA) is a social security benefit that is awarded by the Department of Work and Pensions (formerly the Department of Social Security, or DSS) to disabled people under the age of 65 years to help offset the extra costs of being disabled. There are two components:

- a Mobility Component for people who have difficulty in getting about outdoors,

- a Care Component for people who need the help of another person in performing what are called 'bodily functions', which include such things as dressing, eating, toileting etc.

Claims are made on the basis of self-reporting, which means completing an elaborate claim form that covers every possible aspect of disabling conditions. The claim is assessed by a lay official called a Decision Maker, and a decision is made in the light of information from your doctor and on the basis of entitlement as defined by law. To be entitled to the Mobility Component of DLA you must be either unable or virtually unable to walk. For the Care Component your need for another person to help you with 'bodily functions' should be:

- for a significant part of the day (lowest rate care),
- or frequent attention throughout the day or night (middle rate care),
- or frequent attention throughout the day *and* night (highest rate care).

To qualify for the benefit you have to have had the disabling condition continuously over a period of three months. So you will see that, if you 'only' have periodic attacks, you are very unlikely to be granted a Mobility Component (or the Care Component, for that matter) despite the fact that when an attack is in progress you may be totally unable to walk and be entirely dependent on a carer. In fact, the only circumstances when people with gout might become eligible is the stage of 'chronic tophaceous gout' where a long-term deforming gouty arthritis is present and the disability is such that they are permanently unable (or virtually unable) to walk. The same applies to the Care Component in that you would need the assistance of another person because you are unable to care for yourself independently. Fortunately, in this day and age such circumstances are rare.

For people of 65 years or over, DLA is not applicable but an alternative benefit, Attendance Allowance (AA), is available. This is similar to DLA except that in AA there is no Mobility Component.

This is necessarily a very much abbreviated and simplified account of DLA and AA, which are very complicated benefits. But you can see that, for the most part, gout is not a condition that is likely to be eligible for them, except in rare circumstances.

I am the only daughter in the family, and, although I look in regularly on my elderly father, I don't feel I should be asked to give up my full-time job to look after him when he has a gouty attack. Can't we get a part-time nurse through the social services?

If gout is your father's sole problem, we doubt very much whether it is necessary for you to give up your job in order to look after him. We suspect that he may have other illnesses associated with old age, such as heart failure and/or diabetes. His GP is the best person to judge whether he needs nursing care. Furthermore, the GP can arrange for the services of a community nurse if it is necessary.

With the GP's advice, you could apply for Attendance Allowance (see the previous answer) on his behalf, and find a nursing agency that can supply help when he has an acute attack. It's in your interests to encourage your father to eat and drink sensibly in order to keep down the frequency of attacks.

I quite often suffer from gouty attacks giving a nagging pain in my feet – enough to limit my mobility as a teacher. I get around by having a couple of pairs of special shoes, and I have bought a car with automatic transmission, which involves less movement of my left foot. However, this costs money, just so that I can get to work! Surely there must be some compensation for this?

Disabled Person's Tax Credit is payable when a person loses a job or is forced to accept a lower-paid job because of a disability. It does not seem that this benefit (or Income Support) will be available to you but it is worth discussing the situation at your local Citizens Advice Bureau.

Even with the drugs and careful management of his diet, my husband's gout symptoms are sometimes too bad for him to report to the building site where he works. Can we claim any kind of allowance to help the family income when he can't work?

If someone is unable to work because of illness or disability, Incapacity Benefit is available. Most salaried employees will have a period of six months on statutory sick pay before Incapacity Benefit is payable. If statutory sick pay is not available (this probably applies to your husband if he takes on casual or short-term contracts), Incapacity Benefit starts after three days away from work. Claims must be supported by a certificate from the GP. As with Disability Living Allowance and Attendance Allowance (discussed in the answers above), the award is made by a Department of Work and Pensions (DWP) decision maker, who can require a medical examination undertaken by a DWP-appointed doctor. With certain severe disabilities the person is exempt from undergoing the medical examination.

I have just been diagnosed with primary gout, which I understand is a long-term condition. Must I now declare it to my private health insurance firm?

It is always wise to declare all your medical conditions (including pre-existing conditions) when completing a private healthcare insurance form. Failure to do so may be considered an infringement of the terms of the policy and could result in the forfeiture of benefits. Both acute gouty arthritis and chronic tophaceous gout are treatable conditions and so insurance companies would normally cover their treatment. However, if it began (its 'onset') before you started the policy, the gout may well be excluded. That is to say, you will be covered for any other (non-excluded) condition, but not for any problem directly connected with the gout. Consult the insurance company's helpline, or an insurance broker, as each insurer may have a different approach.

3

Drugs to combat the pain and inflammation

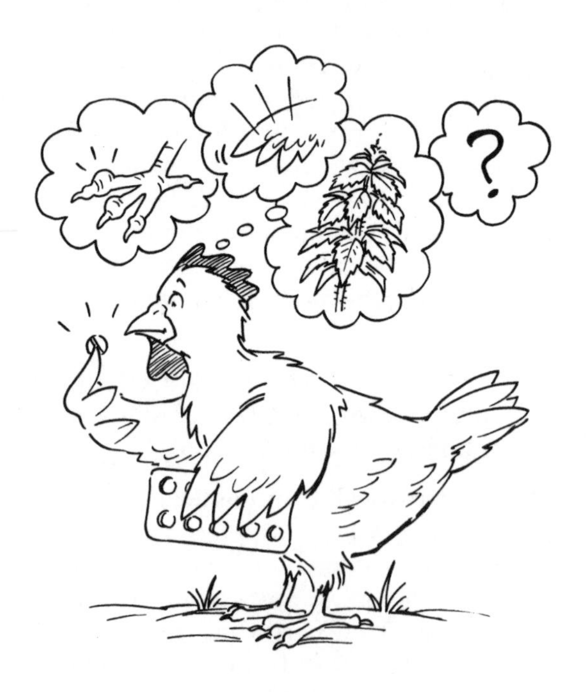

Anyone with personal experience of gout knows that the first indication is an excruciatingly painful episode of 'arthritis', occurring without warning, and sometimes waking them in the early hours of the morning. Modern treatment of the first attack concentrates on these symptoms, and usually relieves the pain and swelling in a short time. Your doctor may prescribe either colchicine or high doses of non-steroidal anti-inflammatory drugs

(NSAIDs); if these don't help enough, they can be followed by an injection of corticosteroids into the affected joint. Occasionally, when all else fails, it may be necessary to use corticosteroids by mouth in tablet form or even by injection into a muscle.

Colchicine

My aunt's GP has given her colchicine. I seem to have heard of it somewhere but not as a medicine. What is colchicine?

We can regard colchicine either as a vindication for 'alternative' medicine or as a triumph for pharmacology! It is an extract from the autumn crocus, *Colchicum autumnale* (see Figure 3.1), which has pale purple flowers in the autumn. You may see the flowers growing in the grass on the Alps or in St James's Park, London, in September. The UK National Collection of *Colchicum* plants is at the National Trust property, Felbrigg Hall, Norfolk. Colchicine has a number of useful effects – but can also be toxic in high doses. (The plants themselves are toxic to grazing animals.) In the controlled doses used for gout, it seems to prevent invasion of the joint by the inflammatory cells, thus also relieving the pain. It should be given within the first 12 hours of the attack if it is to be effective in acute gout. This is only a temporary remedy because your aunt still has to get rid of the excess uric acid from her joints in the longer term.

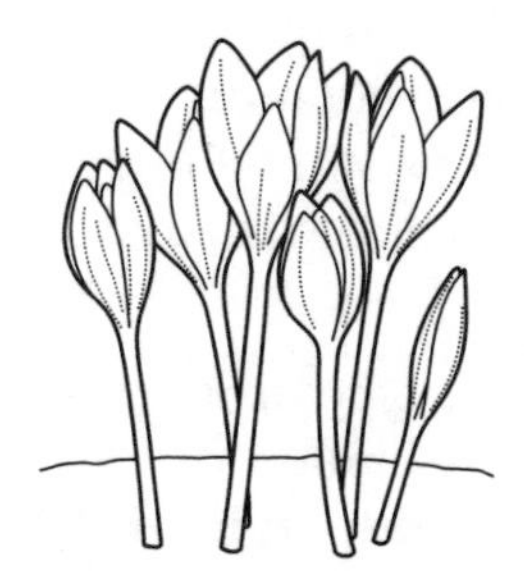

Figure 3.1 Flowers of the autumn crocus.
The drug colchicine is made from this plant, *Colchicum autumnale.*

My doctor gave me colchicine but I seem to be intolerant to it. Are there any alternatives?

When taken by mouth, colchicine causes diarrhoea in many people. It can also be given by injection into the veins but this is hazardous because it may upset the heart rhythm. The alternative is to use NSAIDs (see Table 3.1), which generally do not cause diarrhoea.

Apart from diarrhoea, are there any other hazards connected with the use of colchicine?

Colchicine should never be given to a woman who is or may be pregnant. The drug affects the multiplication of cells, so the developing baby could be affected. Small amounts of colchicine have been found in other herbal extracts; for example, in a formulation of gingko biloba, which has recently been shown to cause defects in babies whose mothers used it regularly during their pregnancy.

I have heard that colchicine can be given between attacks as well as during an attack. Why is this?

As well as being effective against acute attacks, colchicine can be used at a low dose (0.25mg twice a day) over the longer term, even indefinitely, as a preventative (prophylactic) drug. Of course, it does not help to reduce the amount of urate in the body and will not stop urate accumulating, so tophi will continue to enlarge. Thus colchicine is not a very efficient treatment for gout, but it may be helpful in people who get side-effects with urate-lowering drugs or who do not wish to take them.

When I searched an American website, I saw a reference to colchicine being prescribed in a combined form with probenecid. Is it any good, and can I get it on the NHS?

There are differences in treatment between countries and this is one example. Probenecid is a drug that increases the excretion of uric acid through the kidneys. It is now used less widely in the UK (see 'Helping the excretion of uric acid' in Chapter 4), and it has not commonly been used in combination with colchicine. The website you looked at may be out of date, or may be describing only one doctor's preferred treatment. Remember that there is no guarantee that information gleaned from the internet is reliable unless it comes from a reputable source such as a government agency or a well-known institute.

Treating the pain

Are there special drugs to treat the pain of gout?

Because the pain arises from inflammation around the joint, acute gouty arthritis responds either to colchicine or to one of the NSAIDs. These drugs relieve inflammation of any kind, being particularly effective in both acute and chronic forms of arthritis. NSAIDs have been used world-wide for four decades. Of those in current use, naproxen, diclofenac and indometacin have been prescribed most frequently for use in gout. Aspirin should never be used, because at normal doses it slows the excretion of uric acid from the kidneys and so can actually tip the balance towards an acute gouty attack. Paradoxically, at very high doses (20 tablets a day – not recommended!) aspirin has a uricosuric action, helping the excretion of uric acid in the urine. Table 3.1 lists the drugs that are often used for acute gout.

What are COX-2 inhibitors? The doctor who writes in my newspaper seems very enthusiastic about them for arthritis pain.

One of the unfortunate aspects of NSAIDs is their tendency to attack the stomach lining. This (unwanted) side-effect may result in irritation ('gastritis') or more serious complications such as ulceration ('gastric ulceration') or bleeding ('haemorrhage') in the stomach. This is because the principal effect of these drugs is to inhibit enzymes called *cyclo-oxygenase 1* (COX-1) and *cyclo-oxygenase 2* (COX-2), which have a stomach-protecting action, so the price one pays for relief of the inflammation is the risk of gastric damage. The COX-2 inhibitors are a new type of NSAID that give less trouble in the stomach than the older inhibitors, and can give rapid relief in gouty arthritis. They are listed at the end of Table 3.1.

I find that paracetamol is not strong enough for the pain and fever in an acute attack. What else can you recommend?

Paracetamol is a weak pain-killer (analgesic) that has the virtue of not irritating or ulcerating the stomach lining. For conditions in which inflammation plays an important part, such as gout, paracetamol (known as acetaminophen in North America) cannot help. You should be using one of the NSAID family of drugs (see Table 3.1) if the pain is really severe, preferably a COX-2 inhibitor, as this kind is less likely to cause problems in the stomach.

I believe that some drugs can affect other drugs that people might also be taking. Are there any combinations of drugs that I should avoid when taking NSAIDs?

When two (or more) drugs are taken during the course of the same day they could react with one another to produce effects that may be harmful to the person taking them. This is called *drug interaction*, and some people may be very susceptible to the effects. For example, NSAIDs may interact with aspirin and other NSAIDs, anti-clotting agents, anti-epilepsy drugs, lithium (a drug used in some psychiatric conditions) and several other drugs. For these purposes, alcohol is regarded as a drug that may interfere with their action, sometimes with serious results.

If you are concerned about the possibility of your anti-gout medication reacting with another current medication, consult your pharmacist, who is best placed to answer your query.

Table 3.1 Pain-killing drugs recommended for acute gout

Class	Subclass	Generic name	Proprietary name	Combination name
analgesic	mild	codeine*		Co-codamol*
				Co-codaprin**
				Solpadeine*
				Solpadol**
				Tylex**
		dihydrocodeine**	DF 118**	Remedeine**
		paracetamol*	Calpol	Benoral**
				Co-codamol*
				Co-proxamol**
				Distalgesic**
				Remedeine**
				Solpadeine*
				Solpadol**
				Tylex**

Class	Subclass	Generic name	Proprietary name	Combination name
	medium	dextropropoxyphene**		Co-proxamol**
				Distalgesic**
				Doloxene**
	strong	buprenorphine**	Temgesic**	
		nefopam**	Acupan**	
		pentazocine**	Fortagesic**	
			Fortral**	
		tramadol**	Tramake Insts**	Dromadol XL**
			Zamadol SR**	
			Zydol SR**	
NSAIDs	COX-1	acemetacin**	Emflex**	
		aspirin**	Caprin**	Benoral**
			Nu-Seals Aspirin**	Co-codaprin**
		azapropazone**	Rheumox**	
		dexketoprofen**	Keral**	

Class	Subclass	Generic name	Proprietary name	Combination name
NSAIDs	COX-1	diclofenac**	Dicloflex**	Arthrotec**
			Diclomax Retard**	
			Volsaid Retard**	
			Volraman**	
			Voltarol**	
		diflunisal**	Dolobid**	
		fenoprofen**	Fenopron**	
		flurbiprofen**	Froben**	
		ibuprofen *	Brufen *	
			Motrin**	
			Fenbid**	
		indometacin**	Flexin Continus**	
			Indocid**	
		ketoprofen**	Oruvail**	
		ketorolac**	Toradol**	

Class	Subclass	Generic name	Proprietary name	Combination name
NSAIDs	COX-1	mefenamic acid**	Ponstan**	
		naproxen**	Naprosyn EC**	Napratec**
			Synflex**	
		piroxicam**	Brexidol**	
			Feldene**	
		sulindac**	Clinoril**	
		tiaprofenic acid**	Surgam SA**	
	COX-2	celecoxib**	Celebrex**	
		etoricoxib**	Arcoxia**	
		nabumetone**	Relifex**	
		rofecoxib**	Vioxx**	

* Over-the-counter drugs   ** Prescription-only drugs

Notes:

1 The list shows the drugs that are often prescribed for gout. It is *not* meant to be exhaustive.
2 Opiate (morphine-like) pain-killing drugs are omitted because they are habit-forming and therefore unsuitable.
3 Preparations used for children have been omitted from the Table, because medication for gout or for severe pain in children should be given only under strict medical supervision.
4 If in doubt, consult your doctor or pharmacist.

I've heard of people getting addicted to pain-killers and I'm worried it might happen to me. Will I get too accustomed to these drugs or, alternatively, will they lose effectiveness?

Pain-killers such as paracetamol or the NSAIDs do not generally lead to *habituation* (the technical term for addiction). That is to say, they continue to perform reliably as effective pain-killers or as anti-inflammatory agents at the same dosage, and you can take repeated courses or even continue to take them for an indefinite period without their losing their effectiveness. The opiate drugs, by contrast, such as morphine, heroin or pethidine, *are* addictive: if they are used frequently, a higher dose is required to achieve the same desired effect. Because of this they are not suitable for the treatment of acute gout.

However, abuse of pain-killers – especially those obtained 'over the counter' (without needing a prescription) at the pharmacy – is becoming more common and you are right to be concerned. Many of the remedies for headaches, coughs and colds that can be easily purchased from pharmacists contain addictive drugs. They include:

- narcotics such as morphine, codeine, tincture of opium;
- stimulants such as caffeine, ephedrine hydrochloride or pseudephedrine hydrochloride;
- antihistamine sedatives such as diphenhydramine hydrochloride or promethazine hydrochloride.

Read the label on the packet carefully; you will often see a warning about keeping to the recommended dose and not taking the medication for more than three days without medical supervision. This is because overdosing on analgesics can damage your liver, and also because there is a danger of becoming 'hooked' on the extra, addictive, ingredient in the formulation. Regard any tablet, capsule or liquid as a potential hazard, especially if it is marked Plus, Max-Strength, Extra, Adult Formula, and so on. Ask your pharmacist if there is a narcotic or stimulant in any pain-killer that you obtain over the counter or on prescription.

Some other over-the-counter drugs may contain pain-killers; for example, Night Nurse contains paracetamol, so it could be very easy to exceed the maximum recommended dose without realising it. The safest course is to read the label each time you buy or take a drug, and don't throw away packaging that contains crucial information.

My GP has put me on anti-inflammatory drugs. How long do I need to be on them?

You can gradually cut out colchicine or NSAIDs as your urate-lowering drugs stabilise the urate levels at a low value or as the attack of gouty arthritis subsides. Keep some on hand, though, in case you have another gouty attack, and consult your doctor if you have frequent or long-lasting episodes of gout.

Co-proxamol used to be very good for me but it seems to have lost its effectiveness. What can I use now?

Unfortunately, the inflammation in gout can be so acute and the pain so severe that analgesic drugs such as co-proxamol are insufficient to control it, and sometimes potent anti-inflammatory agents called NSAIDs (non-steroidal anti-inflammatory drugs; see Table 3.1) will be needed to control the acute attack. Nowadays only in exceptionally severe attacks that are resistant to NSAIDs will it be necessary to take corticosteroids. These can be taken by mouth (usually as prednisolone tablets) for a week or so, or given by injection into the affected joint (e.g. as methylprednisolone acetate). The injection may also be given into muscle tissue from where it has access to the blood stream. Another possibility is ACTH (adrenocorticotrophic hormone), which stimulates your adrenal glands to secrete extra hydrocortisone. It is given by injection into the muscle tissue.

When I was in hospital I was given steroids for my gout and they gave me rapid relief. Why can't I always have them?

Steroids (corticosteroids) are prescribed when NSAIDs are ineffective, for example in a serious acute attack or after an operation. Occasional use is acceptable, but steroids can have cumulative side-effects such as causing high blood pressure and osteoporosis (thinning of the bones, leading to fractures) if they are used repeatedly.

Complementary methods

A cousin swears by meditation. Can I try meditation to help me with the pain?

There is no scientific evidence that meditation has altered the course of hyperuricaemia or gout for the better. However, you may find that you can override the pain of a gouty attack to some extent if you are experienced in meditation. With all complementary techniques, you could try them *in addition* to the treatment prescribed by your doctor, and see if the benefit is enhanced. Meditation, homoeopathy and aromatherapy are examples of popular complementary techniques, which can be soothing and relaxing. They are, however, no substitute for the drug treatment discussed above. So, whatever you do, keep taking the tablets!

Would cannabis be effective for a painful gouty attack? I've heard that it is useful in multiple sclerosis.

You want to smoke a 'joint' to help your joints?! At present in the UK it is illegal to use cannabis, but this position may be relaxed in the future. Rigorous research for relieving the pain in multiple sclerosis suggests that some components extracted from cannabis plants can be useful. In the future, cannabis preparations may be available on prescription for medical conditions.

My health centre has acupuncture to help with migraine. Would acupuncture help the pain in my joints?

Acupuncture works here by blocking the 'gate' of the pain pathway. According to this theory, the signals travelling up the nerve to the brain generated by the acupuncture needle 'block the gate' so that the pain signals cannot get through. There has been no study of its effectiveness in gout pain, but this is not very different from the nettle cure mentioned in the next question – it may work for some people. Note that the acupuncture needles are not necessarily inserted into the site of the inflammation!

I heard something on the radio about the use of stinging nettles in the treatment of arthritis pain – will it be effective against gout?

A research project is in progress to investigate numerous claims that contact from stinging nettles on the skin near an arthritic joint, although causing some pain and inflammation itself, noticeably relieves the pain in the joints over a few days. Many people have reported that this treatment helps their osteoarthritis, but there has been no study of people specifically with gout because they are a small proportion of those with arthritis symptoms. If you are willing and brave enough, try it, and tell your GP if it works!

4

Drugs to lower the level of urate in the blood

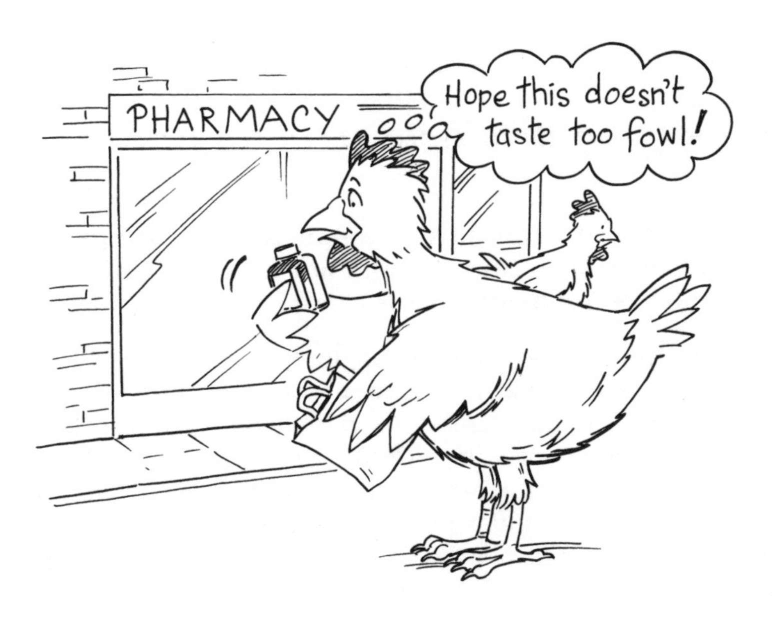

Once the acute attack has been dealt with, you may have a long period without symptoms. Typically 6–12 months may elapse before your next attack of gouty arthritis. You may be asked to visit the rheumatology out-patient clinic and to give regular samples of blood and urine. The clinic will monitor the levels of sodium urate in your blood and urine, to see if you need to take drugs to regulate the concentration of urate in your body fluids.

Your doctor may prescribe drugs such as probenecid, sulfinpyrazone (Anturan) or benzbromarone (Desuric) to help the excretion of uric acid from your kidneys. This action is called *uricosuric* and the drugs are called *uricosuric agents*. You should tell your doctor if you are taking any other drugs or alternative/complementary remedies, because some will affect the ability of your kidneys to excrete uric acid.

The introduction of allopurinol in 1966 was a major advance in the treatment of gout. Allopurinol (Zyloric) inhibits the last step in the production of uric acid from purines. This drug is a valuable help in controlling the rate at which uric acid is made throughout the day from the purines in the body's system.

Measuring uric acid in body fluids

I've been asked to produce a sample for measuring uric acid and have been told I should not have any caffeine for three days beforehand. Why is this?

Caffeine (from coffee) and theophylline and theobromine (from tea) are chemicals that resemble uric acid in structure, and so can interfere with the methods used to identify and measure uric acid in the blood or urine. Coffee and tea are not the only sources: watch out for caffeine in any form of cola, headache pills and cold cures, and in pick-me-up drinks such as Red Bull or Lucozade, all of which will be labelled as containing caffeine. Similar chemicals may be found in herbal teas and in confectionery, desserts or hot drinks containing chocolate.

You will usually be asked to provide both blood and urine, so that a comparison can be made of the urate level in the two fluids. You should be careful not to take vitamin tablets or antibiotics during these few days, or any other drugs or herbal remedies that might affect the way in which uric acid is excreted into the urine. If you are not sure whether something you are taking could be involved in this way, ask your pharmacist or doctor.

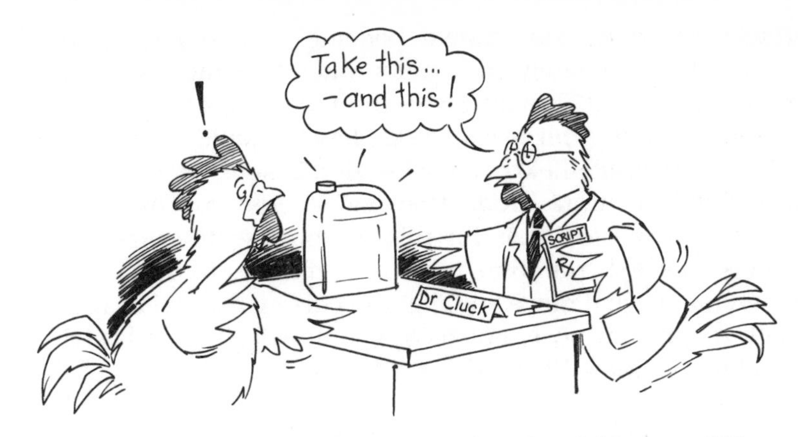

I have been asked to collect my urine for 24 hours. Why does the hospital lab want so much when surely the tests only need a small volume?

Uric acid and other components are excreted at different rates throughout the day – and the first urine of the day is usually the most concentrated. Excretion of uric acid will vary according to when and what you have eaten during the day. To even out all these variables, a 24-hour sample is collected, which will contain the sum of everything that has passed through in that period. The container may seem dauntingly large when you first see it, but you must put all your urine for the day into it: it contains a small amount of preservative (so don't empty it out when you get it home!). The laboratory will measure the volume as well as the contents of the collection. They may warm it slightly to ensure that all the contents are dissolved, and then send a small bottleful to another laboratory for analysis. If your 24-hour sample is a small volume, it will show that you should increase your intake of fluids to flush out all the dissolved components; this means passing at least two litres of urine per day.

I'm now taking urate-lowering drugs. Can I, or should I, have my uric acid level measured regularly?

Once your plasma urate level has settled back into the normal range following the introduction of urate-lowering drugs the attacks of acute gout should become less frequent and less severe, and ultimately may peter out altogether, so that you become gout-free. Provided you continue to take the drugs in the prescribed dose, your plasma urate levels should remain normal, unless there is an unexpected alteration in some factor in the balance between urate production and excretion. The key word here is *unexpected.* It is for this reason that the plasma urate level is checked from time to time, to make sure that it remains within the normal range and that the current dose of drug is adequate for this purpose. For most people whose gout is stable, a blood test every 6–12 months is sufficient.

Is there any hope of home-testing kits for uric acid in the urine or in the blood, like diabetics doing a home test of their blood sugar?

The test for uric acid is based on a reaction that can't be done easily at home, so home-testing is not possible at the moment.

My mother is 70 and she has been taking a diuretic – frusemide – for about 30 years, which she started because she was getting very swollen ankles. Might she be in danger of developing gout? If so, should she ask her doctor to get a measurement of uric acid in her blood?

Diuretic drugs help to remove excess fluid from the body and as such are very widely used in the treatment of diseases such as heart failure or nephrotic syndrome (a kidney complaint in which fluid is retained by the kidneys). One of the side-effects of diuretic drugs such as frusemide is that they cause the kidneys to retain urate. This effect is so potent that it can bring about (or aggravate existing) hyperuricaemia and gout. So, yes, it would be a good idea to check the blood urate level, especially if she has symptoms suggesting gout. At the same time it might be reasonable to question whether, in fact, the diuretic is still required. Unless her ankles swell if she doesn't take it, the obvious solution would be to stop the diuretic drug.

Uric acid and the kidneys

During a gout attack my urine becomes very yellow and smelly. If this is uric acid and the kidneys are working overtime, could I 'flush' the system by drinking lots of water? Can I use the colour of my urine as an early warning?

Urine colour provides a very rough guide to the concentration of dissolved components, and you will be familiar with the normal yellow colour when you are drinking an adequate amount of fluid. If you left your urine in a chamber pot or other container, you might see a reddish deposit of uric acid crystals. People with kidney stones are generally advised to have a two-litre bottle of water with them, and to drink the contents during the day *in addition to* other beverages. Even those in no danger of developing kidney stones should be passing at least two litres of urine every day, the fluid for which will have come from food, especially fruit and vegetables, as well as from drinking. Clearly you need to look closely at how much fluid you take in during the day, and keep yourself topped up with water. It can be mineral water or tap water, cold or hot.

I already have to get up several times in the night to pass urine, and I dread drinking any more fluid.

If you are a middle-aged or older man, you should be looking out for problems with your prostate, a gland that surrounds the urine-bearing passage in your groin. The first signs of trouble are the need to pass urine frequently, because an enlarged prostate restricts how much the bladder can contain and prevents it from emptying completely. If you feel that this might apply to you, ask your doctor to investigate for PSA (prostate-specific antigen) in your blood and to check that your prostate is healthy and that your bladder is working properly.

I have gout and I wonder if I am likely to get uric acid kidney stones as well. If so, how can the risk be minimised?

Uric acid stones form in the kidneys of people who have a lifestyle, diet or metabolism that leads to the following risk factors:

- a high level of uric acid in the urine,
- highly acid urine (connected with exercise and with the excretion of other components of the diet),
- a low volume of urine,
- significant loss of fluid in perspiration (e.g. people living in a hot climate, or taking strenuous exercise),
- a combination of these factors.

A diet that is high in meat, fish or poultry is particularly bad in this respect as it leads to a high level of uric acid *and* acidic urine. The general rules are to drink a lot of water, and don't take too much salt with your food or eat too many salty snacks. By passing at least two litres of urine a day, you will help to prevent the formation of stones made up of the less-soluble components.

The doctor has told me that I need to make my urine less acidic (more alkaline). Why is this?

If you are seeing a specialist for the treatment of kidney stones, you may have been prescribed sodium bicarbonate or potassium citrate. This treatment aims to increase the pH value of your urine to about 6.5 in a 24-hour urine sample. A pH value lower than 5.4 indicates extreme acidity, and will prevent the uric acid from dissolving in your urine. There is a great risk that conditions favouring acidic urine will lead to a build-up of stones in your kidneys. Sodium bicarbonate (baking soda, also found in the pain-killer Beecham's Powders) is effective but it tends to increase the excretion of calcium, which is needed for bones and teeth. Potassium citrate is better, but in the UK it is only provided as a liquid that tastes unpleasant unless it is mixed with a flavoured drink such as orange juice.

It is such a performance to take a urine sample to the hospital for testing. Can I check the acidity of my urine at home?

The acidity of your urine will be measured along with tests for other contents, so it is important that you give samples to the hospital laboratory. However, you can do a simple test at home. The principle is exactly the same as the litmus paper you may remember using in school chemistry classes to measure acidity. The widely available Dipstix papers, as well as testing for protein, glucose and blood, also give an approximate pH reading when the paper is dipped in a specimen of freshly passed urine. You can buy Dipstix from all dispensing chemist shops.

I've often seen cranberry juice mentioned in magazines for helping to keep bladder infections away. Would fruit juices have any use in helping the excretion of uric acid?

Cranberry juice is often recommended for people with urinary tract infections, as it seems to be the only fruit juice that actually acidifies urine enough to prevent the growth of bacteria in the bladder. Unfortunately, this acidifying effect would promote the formation of uric acid stones in the urinary tract, especially if you have a high rate of uric acid excretion and/or a low volume of urine. So you should avoid cranberry juice, but other fruit juices are all right in moderation.

I have problems emptying my bladder because of an enlarged prostate. Does this have implications for my gout, which has troubled me a few times in the last five years?

It sounds as though you have developed some obstruction to the flow of urine out of the bladder as a result of the enlargement of your prostate. Anything that obstructs the passage of urine will increase the risk of forming bladder stones, and uric acid bladder stones are fairly common in older men with an enlarged prostate. This is partly because urine tends to become more acidic as we get older, and partly from the retention of urine as the bladder fails to empty completely when passing urine. This is likely to affect your gout only when the obstruction causes enough 'back-pressure' to damage the kidneys. If the kidneys deteriorate, the plasma urate level begins to climb and may threaten further attacks of gout. The problem should be sorted out if you have an operation to relieve or remove the obstruction.

Helping the excretion of uric acid

I don't like to take drugs unless it's really necessary. How do drugs help the kidneys excrete uric acid efficiently?

There is a balance between excretion and reabsorption of soluble components as urine is made in the kidneys. Uric acid goes back into the blood and is constantly recycled unless it is deposited as crystals in joints or as insoluble stones in the kidneys. Uricosuric drugs (and some antibiotics) help by pushing the balance towards excretion of uric acid in your urine, and this lowers the concentration in your blood.

I have heard that the uricosuric drug probenecid has been withdrawn and thus is no longer available in the UK. This drug has kept my gout at bay for 30 years. What do you advise me to do?

The situation is not quite as gloomy as you think. It is true that the production of Benemid, the brand of probenecid marketed by Merck Sharpe & Dohme for half a century, although still licensed in the UK, has been discontinued for marketing reasons. (This is a polite way of saying there was no money in it!) The good news is that a generic (non-branded) probenecid imported from Sweden is available on prescription from your GP on a 'named-patient basis'. If you take the prescription to your pharmacy/chemist shop, they can obtain the drug for you direct from the importers, IDIS World Medicines (see Appendix 1, ***Useful addresses***, for contact details).

I am taking uricosuric drugs to help excrete uric acid in my urine. Are they only available by prescription?

Uricosuric drugs are listed in Table 4.1 and you will see that the choice is very limited. Your pharmacist will have a little more trouble getting hold of probenecid or benzbromarone if your GP prefers to prescribe either of them. They are available only on prescription.

If I take uricosuric drugs, will they affect any other medicine I may be taking?

Because they increase the filtration of uric acid through the kidneys, uricosuric drugs also increase the rate at which some other drugs are lost from the body through this route. Bronchodilators (for asthma) containing aminophylline or theophylline are less effective when used with uricosuric drugs. In contrast, probenecid inhibits the excretion of penicillin, several other antibiotics and the cancer drug methotrexate, so their dose should be reduced if you are already taking probenecid. Always keep your doctor informed of any preparation or drug that you may be taking, including herbal remedies.

Other examples that may 'antagonise' the action of uricosuric drugs are:

- aspirin and another anti-inflammatory drug phenylbutazone,
- diuretics such as thiazides (e.g. amiloride, bendrofluazide, chlortalidone, cyclopenthiazide),
- loop diuretics (e.g. frusemide), taken for heart disease, high blood pressure (hypertension) or puffy ankles (oedema),
- pyrazinamide, an anti-tuberculosis drug,
- high doses of the vitamins niacin (B_3) or nicotinic acid.

Table 4.1 Uricosuric drugs used in the treatment of gout and hyperuricaemia

Generic name	Proprietary name	Usual dosage	Comments
benzbromarone	Desuric	100–200mg/day	Effective for severe tophaceous gout and in the presence of kidney damage. Officially not licensed in the UK but available through chemists on NHS or private prescription on a 'named-patient basis'. Can be obtained by pharmacists from John Bell & Croyden, IDIS World Medicines or Welbeck Pharmaceuticals & Hospital Supplies (contact details in Appendix 1, ***Useful addresses***).
probenecid	Benuryl (ICN,Canada) Probecid (Astra, Sweden) Probenecid Medic (Denmark) Probenecid Weimar (Germany)	1–2g/day	No longer distributed in the UK but available on NHS or private prescription on a 'named-patient basis' through pharmacies. Can be obtained by pharmacists from IDIS World Medicines or Welbeck Pharmaceuticals & Hospital Supplies (contact details in Appendix 1, ***Useful addresses***)
sulfinpyrazone	Anturan	200–600mg/day	Available only on prescription. Less effective in the presence of kidney damage.

Apart from vitamins and aspirin, all of these will be prescribed by your doctor, whom you should tell about any and all other treatments that you are taking.

I've been considering taking an aspirin every day, as it has been recommended to prevent heart attacks, deep vein thrombosis and strokes in middle-aged and older people, but now I hear that aspirin counteracts the effects of uricosuric drugs. Is this a problem at the low doses I was planning to use?

There is very good evidence that a daily dose of 75mg of aspirin – equivalent to one junior aspirin tablet – prevents clot formation (thrombosis) in blood vessels, and if you have been recommended to take it you should certainly do so. There is, though, a small possibility that the aspirin may cause your kidneys to retain a little more urate than previously, resulting in a rise in your plasma urate level. So it is a good idea for your blood to be tested from time to time, to check that the urate level is still under control. If it is not, it may be necessary to adjust your uricosuric drug or allopurinol a little. Discuss this point with your doctor.

If caffeine is a diuretic and also resembles uric acid, why is it all right for me to drink coffee?

There are several answers to this question. Although the caffeine molecule is similar to uric acid, its breakdown products are more soluble and so it is excreted readily from the kidneys, unless taken in very large quantities. Coffee, tea and cola drinks are so widely available that it would be difficult to imagine cutting them out completely but, because they are stimulants and habit-forming, it is probably wise to limit them to about three cups (or glasses) per day.

Diuretics such as coffee, alcohol and concentrated fruit drinks cause the loss of water through the kidneys – and can lead to 'net dehydration' even though you are taking in adequate amounts of fluid. In addition, coffee provides a significant proportion of the daily requirement of nicotinic acid (niacin, or vitamin B_3), so very large quantities of coffee might provide enough niacin to cause the kidneys to retain more urate instead of excreting it. All of these are good reasons for cutting down the amount of coffee and replacing it with water.

I would rather not take chemicals, which is how I regard drugs. Has any complementary medicine been shown to help the body excrete uric acid?

Health food shops may suggest nettle leaves (Latin name: *Urtica dioica*) in the form of tablets or an infusion (a drink made with hot water) to enhance the excretion of uric acid. You may find that regular use is helpful but it is important not to give up on the prescription drugs. Most of the other alternative treatments offered for 'kidney ailments' are diuretics and thus cause the body to retain uric acid.

Vitamin C (ascorbic acid) at high doses is known to help the excretion of uric acid, when used without prescribed uricosuric drugs. These doses may also encourage diarrhoea, however, which could cause an overall loss of fluid from the body.

Many GPs are sympathetic to your opinion and some are trained in complementary medicine, so it is worthwhile your discussing this when your doctor offers to prescribe drugs for you. You should be aware that complementary remedies may cost you more than the prescription drugs for the same condition, and of course you must tell your doctor if you are taking both kinds of treatment, as one may interact unexpectedly with another. Do be wary about using herbal remedies, whether Chinese or Western. The strength and purity of the products can vary according to where the plant is grown and the stage at which it is harvested; there have been reports of serious illness and even death resulting from someone taking a herbal remedy. Similarly, confirm that the therapist is fully trained to recommend the appropriate treatment.

I was very excited to read in a health magazine about a herbal remedy that acts in the same way as gout drugs. Would it be a reasonable alternative to allopurinol?

You have probably read about Quercetin, which can be bought in capsule form at health food shops. It is a flavonoid, a coloured compound obtained from the leaves of plants (and therefore also found in leafy vegetables and tea). It has some effect against inflammation but it also prevents the action of xanthine oxidase, thus acting like allopurinol (as explained in the next section). The only problem is that extracts of plant material may not be as well standardised as synthetic drugs such as allopurinol, so you may get a variable response to regular doses of Quercetin. If you were to take Quercetin and allopurinol, you would need to use a smaller dose of the latter, so be sure to tell your doctor if you decide to try this herbal remedy.

Controlling the formation of uric acid

My GP says that I must take a drug to control the formation of uric acid. Which is the best one, and how does it work?

Allopurinol is the best drug for controlling the formation of uric acid. It acts by blocking the enzyme that converts the purine breakdown products hypoxanthine or xanthine to uric acid. However, xanthine is even more insoluble than uric acid, and so it must not be allowed to accumulate to a higher concentration, because it too can form kidney stones. The concentration of xanthine in the urine can be measured at a specialist unit, and if it is approaching its solubility limit, the dose of allopurinol will need to be reduced. On a day-to-day basis, people with most forms of primary and secondary gout can help themselves by limiting the amount of purine-rich food in their diet (see Chapter 5, ***Food and drink***), and by taking allopurinol regularly as prescribed by their doctor.

Extremely high levels of sodium urate may accumulate in a person with a metabolic disorder (see Chapter 6, ***Gout in young***

people). In such a case, the dose of allopurinol must be monitored very carefully to prevent the kidneys from being damaged by the accumulation of xanthine.

After a week in hospital for a bad attack of gastroenteritis, my elderly mother found that her feet were too painful to walk on. Although the problem was diagnosed as gout or podagra, I was very surprised that they didn't immediately start her on allopurinol, which I know is the gout drug. Why was this?

If this was her first attack of gouty arthritis, the doctor was right to avoid using allopurinol in the acute stage. This would cause a sudden lowering of uric acid levels, which might trigger a new attack or extend the existing attack. Your mother will have been given colchicine and NSAIDs to deal with the pain and inflammation. Then allopurinol would be prescribed to reduce her urate levels after the attack had subsided.

The doctor has put me on allopurinol. How long will I have to take it?

The first few prescriptions may run for a short period, such as a month, because your doctor will want to see you fairly frequently until the symptoms have stabilised. After that, you will probably pick up a three-month supply with each prescription. Even when your plasma urate level reaches normal values, you will continue to take allopurinol indefinitely. For most people this means for life.

Should I take my allopurinol with food, or all in one go when I get up in the morning?

Most people take a single 300mg tablet first thing every day. However, you may be advised to take allopurinol in 'divided doses' and with food. This is very convenient if you have a regular schedule for eating your meals, as each occasion will remind you to drink a glass of water and take an allopurinol tablet.

I take allopurinol regularly. Should I keep up the normal dose when I have an acute attack of podagra?

Yes, keep taking it as normal. Stopping allopurinol if you have an acute attack of podagra will have the inevitable effect of a further rise in the plasma urate level, which will increase the likelihood of further acute attacks in the near future or cause the present attack to last longer.

My joints are actually more painful and inflamed than before I started on drugs. Can I stop taking the allopurinol?

For the first few months of urate-lowering drug therapy (with either uricosuric drugs or allopurinol) there is always a tendency for the acute gout problem to get worse (exacerbate). The drug causes a rapid decline in the total amount of urate in the body fluids and tissues, but there may also be major fluctuations in the level of urate in and around the joints. As the level in the surrounding fluid falls there is a tendency for some crystals to re-dissolve, leading to uneven distribution of urate in the blood plasma, including some isolated pockets where the concentration may be high enough to allow new crystals or deposits to be laid down.

The general trend, however, is a fall in urate levels, and so you should persevere with the treatment. This tendency to develop acute attacks usually peters out within 6–12 months.

I haven't had an attack of gouty arthritis for some time now. Can I gradually take less allopurinol?

The fact that you have stopped getting attacks of gout suggests that your plasma urate level is being adequately controlled (i.e. is being held within the normal range), and this is how it should be. If you reduce your current dose of allopurinol, the plasma urate level will slowly begin to rise and with it the risk of further attacks of gout ensuing. So if you are tempted to stop or reduce the dose of allopurinol because you have stopped getting attacks of gout, please don't be rash. You may regret it!

Diet and allopurinol

I stopped drinking beer when the doctor told me that it was contributing to my gout. Can I drink beer again now that I am taking allopurinol?

You would be wise to be cautious about resuming beer drinking. Strictly speaking, once your gout treatment has stabilised (i.e. the plasma urate level is normalised and you have stopped having acute attacks) you may eat small amounts of purine-rich foods (and drink beer) in strict moderation without the risk of provoking further attacks of gout. But take care! Alcohol in general, and especially when drunk without food, has a specific effect that promotes the retention of urate by the kidneys.

See Chapter 5 (***Food and drink***) for more on the topic of diet.

I know that I must watch my diet. But when a special occasion is coming up, can't I just take a bit more allopurinol than normal, like diabetics who adjust their insulin intake?

Urate levels in the blood can rise in response to excessive purine intake – for example, if you eat a rich meal. However, urate levels do not fluctuate as widely or as rapidly as the blood sugar level does, nor does allopurinol act as rapidly on urate as insulin does to lower the sugar in the blood. Consequently, there is less need for 'fine tuning' of the dose of allopurinol. So there is no point in taking extra allopurinol in anticipation of a 'binge', whether it is of food or drink. Just don't 'go off the rails' too often.

Will loss of appetite – for example, when I have a cold or flu – affect the amount of allopurinol I should take?

It is important for to you to take the same dose of your prescribed drug, be it a uricosuric drug or allopurinol, day in, day out. This is regardless of how you feel, whatever your appetite, or whether you have another illness such as a cold or flu. It is extremely important to maintain a good volume of urine, so you should drink more water when you feel feverish. Only in this way will you maintain your plasma urate in a constant satisfactory (and normal) level, thereby ensuring that you do not drift back into a tendency to get gout attacks.

I don't really like taking drugs. Could I just try to eat sensibly and not otherwise treat the gout with allopurinol?

You can make a huge difference to your general health – and to the gout symptoms – by cutting down on calories, purines and beer. Measures that help fight heart disease, high blood pressure and diabetes – switching away from animal fats, salt and sugar – will also pay off against the painful wear on your joints. You might be one of a small number of people with infrequent attacks of primary gout or a mildly raised urate level who can succeed with a low-purine diet alone, but do consider taking allopurinol regularly if you start to get attacks again.

Long-term allopurinol treatment

After 15 years, allopurinol doesn't seem to be effective any more. Although I try to eat a low-purine diet, I have started to have gouty attacks much more frequently. Is this normal?

No, it is most unusual. Allopurinol does not tend to lose its effect over time no matter how many years you take it. There are several possible explanations for your problem:

- Your need for allopurinol may have increased for some reason, such as a change in diet or exercise. Checking the plasma urate to see if it has risen into the hyperuricaemic range will confirm this state of affairs. If so, your doctor will want to raise your allopurinol dose until the urate level has fallen again.

- You are not taking the correct dose as prescribed by the doctor. Check the label on the bottle to make sure that you have not forgotten the correct dose or how often you should take it. The most common cause for the 'failure of allopurinol' is failure on the part of the person to take the drug correctly!
- It may be that an unrelated kidney disease or the introduction of an additional drug such as a diuretic or an NSAID has damaged the ability of your kidneys to excrete uric acid. Either of these drugs may tip the balance in favour of retention rather than excretion of uric acid. In such situations a combination of allopurinol and benzbromarone is helpful.

I've developed a skin rash and I feel distinctly unwell when I take allopurinol. My GP thinks I may be allergic to the drug – what does this mean? Can I take other drugs that work in the same way?

Allergy is an immune reaction whereby the body reacts to a substance in an exaggerated or violent way. This usually takes the form of a rash, which is uncomfortable but otherwise not serious. However, in some people, the reaction may affect the liver and kidneys, and may even become life-threatening. If this is the case with you and the allopurinol, you cannot keep on with the drug; continuing to do so would be highly dangerous. It should be stressed that such allergies are extremely rare; allopurinol is consumed daily world-wide without ill-effect.

There are a number of options available to tackle this situation:

1. There is a method of 'desensitising' a person who is allergic to allopurinol. It is a slow, tedious and uncertain approach, which is not recommended except perhaps in the mildest type of allergic reaction. It involves starting with a minute dose of the drug and then slowly and steadily doubling it until the usual therapeutic dose is achieved, hoping all the time that there is no allergic reaction, which would bring the exercise to an abrupt end.
2. Substitute probenecid or sulfinpyrazone for the allopurinol;

they are both uricosuric drugs well established in the treatment of hyperuricaemia and gout. Caution is needed, though, if you have a tendency to form uric acid kidney stones, for fear of adding to the urate load borne by your kidneys and risking promoting kidney failure.

3 Substitute benzbromarone for the allopurinol. This is a powerful uricosuric drug, particularly useful in treating people with gout who are allergic to allopurinol. It is effective even in people with severe gout, including those who have kidney impairment (which is not the usual case with uricosuric drugs) and/or those with tophaceous gout, but the risk of urate stones still applies, as in point 2. See Table 4.1 for the wholesalers who can supply your pharmacist with this drug.

I believe that some medicines don't work well when taken together. Are there any drugs I shouldn't take with allopurinol?

Some drugs given in the treatment of cancerous diseases and some used to treat certain so-called autoimmune rheumatic diseases such as SLE (systemic lupus erythematosus) or rheumatoid arthritis may cause a problem. Of these, the most widely used are azathioprine (widely used to treat severe rheumatic diseases) and cyclosporine (used to suppress the body's immune system after organ transplantation). Allopurinol should be used with caution when taken at the same time as these drugs, as it enhances their action. Their dose should be reduced to between one-third and one-quarter when being taken as well as allopurinol.

My wife has been taking allopurinol since she developed gout in her late teens. We want to start a family and I am worried about her continuing to take allopurinol during the pregnancy.

Gout is most unusual in young women, so your wife should first get advice on whether she has a metabolic disorder, which her children are thus likely to inherit. She may need to give blood and urine samples for her GP to send to a specialist centre for analysis (see Chapter 6, ***Gout in young people***).

You and your wife should decide what to do after discussion with your doctor. Most doctors would be reluctant to prescribe either allopurinol or uricosuric drugs (or even NSAIDs) to a pregnant woman, out of concern that they might damage the unborn baby. However, we know of twin sisters with a condition called familial juvenile hyperuricaemic nephropathy (FJHN; see Chapter 6), who continued their allopurinol throughout pregnancy in the 1970s. Their children were unaffected by the allopurinol.

On the other hand, it is very important that pregnant women should not take colchicine or any herbal remedy that might contain it, because it has been proved to damage the development of the baby.

What are the long-term consequences if I decide not to take allopurinol, but just rely on anti-inflammatories to get me through the attacks of gouty arthritis?

You might get away with it if your urate levels remain reasonably normal! If, however, your urate levels remain high (either because of a purine-rich diet or because of natural over-production of purines) and you decide that you don't want to take allopurinol, you are likely to develop successive attacks of acute gout and the intervals between them will gradually become shorter. You may have the misfortune to suffer increasingly severe and protracted attacks. As the months go by, more and more urate may be deposited in and around your joints and in your tissues. These deposits may begin to cause damage to adjacent bone, which will become eroded, resulting in deformities (especially foot deformities) developing and causing difficulty in walking. You may start to limp and require a walking stick (even a wheelchair!). Untreated tophaceous gout is not a pleasant disease. Are you sure that you prefer not to accept allopurinol, which can prevent all this from happening?

5

Food and drink

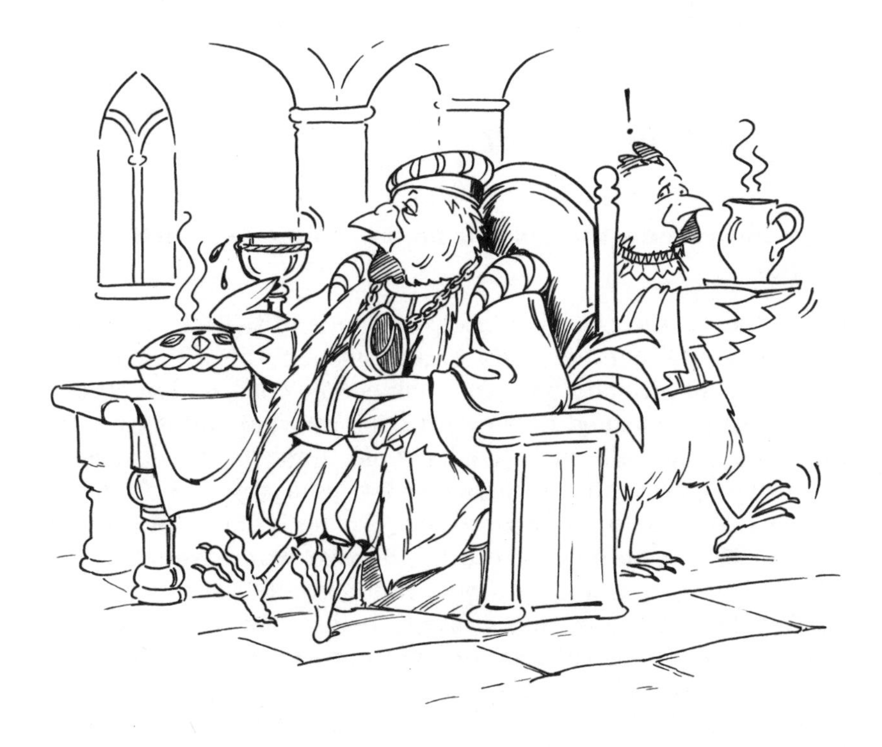

We seem to be bombarded with information about our diet nowadays. Numerous articles in magazines and newspapers advise us to eat less fat (especially saturated fat from animals) and to increase the amount of fruit and vegetables in our diet. Most of us should also eat fewer calories and take more exercise to lose weight and increase our physical fitness, and this is especially true if we wish to reduce the strain on arthritic joints.

Gout is the only form of arthritis whose symptoms can definitely be helped through diet. No expensive ingredients or food supplements are required. Simply cutting calories can help most people with primary gout, but most important of all is to limit foods containing high concentrations of purines. In this chapter we provide you with a list of these foods. Some people report that gouty attacks are triggered by other foods (such as strawberries, citrus fruit or tomatoes) that are not high in purines. If you find that these foods cause you trouble, cut them out too.

Eating like a king

How do we know that classic gout is connected with what we eat?

First, there is the clear historical evidence of the well-fed, middle-aged gouty men beloved by cartoonists in the 17th and 18th centuries. An ordinary meal for such people consisted of several meat courses, washed down with copious wine and spirits. On the other hand, although most people drank beer because of fears of contaminated drinking water, gout was not found in poorer people with a restricted diet. Secondly, cases of primary gout were very infrequent during the two world wars in 20th-century Europe, when food was rationed and very little meat was available. As food supplies returned to normal, and indeed as the population began to eat better than ever before, gout (and obesity) became much more common among older men.

During the second half of the 20th century, a wide-ranging analysis of the chemical constituents of foodstuffs highlighted a direct link between a diet rich in purines and their role in triggering a gouty attack in susceptible people.

I've read somewhere that Henry VIII had gout. Is this so?

The well-known portraits of an overweight middle-aged Henry VIII certainly suggest that he enjoyed eating and drinking, both of which are risk factors for gout because they can lead to increasingly high levels of uric acid in the blood (hyperuricaemia) over several years. Other risk factors are high blood pressure (hypertension) and Type 2 diabetes (the 'adult' form), which we regard as diseases of plenty, as they are prevalent in the West. Most Western people today eat a diet that would have been regarded as rich by Henry's subjects; they could only dream of eating meat and drinking wine every day but, as long as their meagre diet kept them alive, they were unlikely to suffer from gout. Hence gout has been known as the 'king of diseases and the disease of kings'.

To answer your question, Henry VIII had a number of problems – among them syphilis, which can cause arthritis – and textbooks say that he had gout, too. Unfortunately, we cannot test him for high urate levels to confirm the diagnosis!

The Prince Regent (who became King George IV) definitely had gout. He was racked with pain until, in 1817, he gratefully began to use extracts of colchicum, an ancient remedy that had recently been accepted again by medical opinion.

I've been putting on a bit of weight. Does being overweight make my gout symptoms worse?

If you are overweight, you should definitely try to cut the total amount of food you eat, to decrease the load placed on your joints, especially on your knees and feet. A high body weight arises from eating more than your body needs to keep going, and the excess is stored as fat.

Several factors are relevant if you are overweight and have primary gout. Overweight and obese people run the risk of developing hypertension and Type 2 diabetes, all of which can put extra stress on the kidneys and reduce the ability of the kidneys to excrete uric acid. Reducing your weight to the 'healthy' range also helps to lower the concentration of uric acid in the plasma, thus reducing the risks of crystals being deposited in the joints.

Is there a difference between being overweight and being obese?

Depending on your height, there is a range of healthy weights within which you have a much lower risk of developing heart disease, Type 2 diabetes, hypertension and primary gout. The Body Mass Index (BMI), calculated from height and weight, has a value of 20–25 in this 'healthy' range. Values of 25–30 are 'overweight', 30–40 are 'obese', and above 40 is 'dangerously obese'. These figures are shown in Figure 5.1, and you can read off your height (in metres) against your weight (in kilograms), noting in which zone the combined values fall.

However, we need to use some common sense when considering weight! Muscle mass is very dense, and some people who are extremely physically fit may have BMI values in the 'overweight' or 'obese' range. Serious conditions such as Type 2 diabetes and heart disease are associated with deposits of fat around the middle of the body, so it is equally important to consider one's shape, or the relationship of waist, hip and height measurements. Dr Margaret Ashwell, a leading nutrition scientist, believes that it is wrong to rely on the BMI when deciding whether you are overweight and she has developed the Ashwell chart (Figure 5.2). Fat deposits can be measured using skin-fold callipers (at a gym or health centre) or you can simply measure your waist – men with a waist measurement above 94cm are at increased risk, as are women with a waist measurement greater than 80cm; and those above 102cm (men) or 88cm (women) are at a significantly increased risk of disease related to obesity.

Watching what I eat is so boring, and I find it hard to stick to a strict diet. Is there a quick and easy way to lose weight?

Almost every magazine for women – and several designed for men – contains detailed diets for weight loss, especially between the New Year and the summer holidays. If these regimens were easy to follow, and guaranteed success, we would not need to see them again and again each year. Faddy diets, for example those

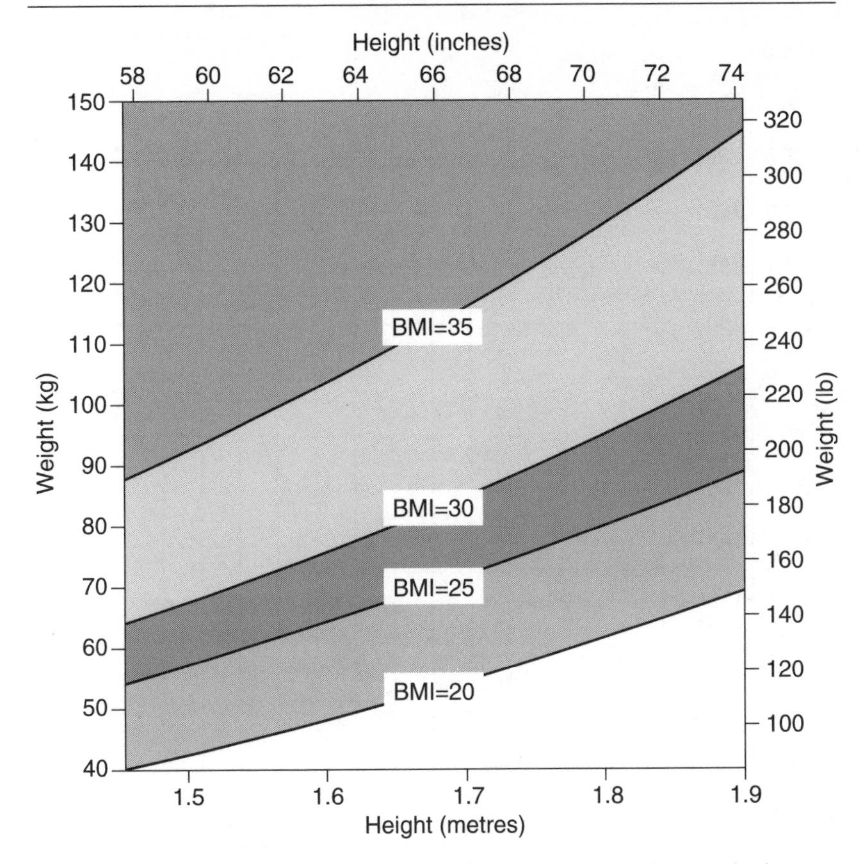

Figure 5.1 The body mass index (BMI) chart. Use the chart or do the calculation below to find out your BMI: divide your weight in kilograms by the square of your height in metres.

Your BMI score:
below 20: underweight
20–25: ideal
25–30: overweight
30+: seriously overweight

$$\text{BMI} = \frac{\text{weight in kilograms}}{(\text{height in metres})^2}$$

For example, if you weigh 70 kg and are 1.7 metres tall, your BMI will be:

$$\frac{70}{(1.7)^2} = \frac{70}{(2.9)} = 24.1$$

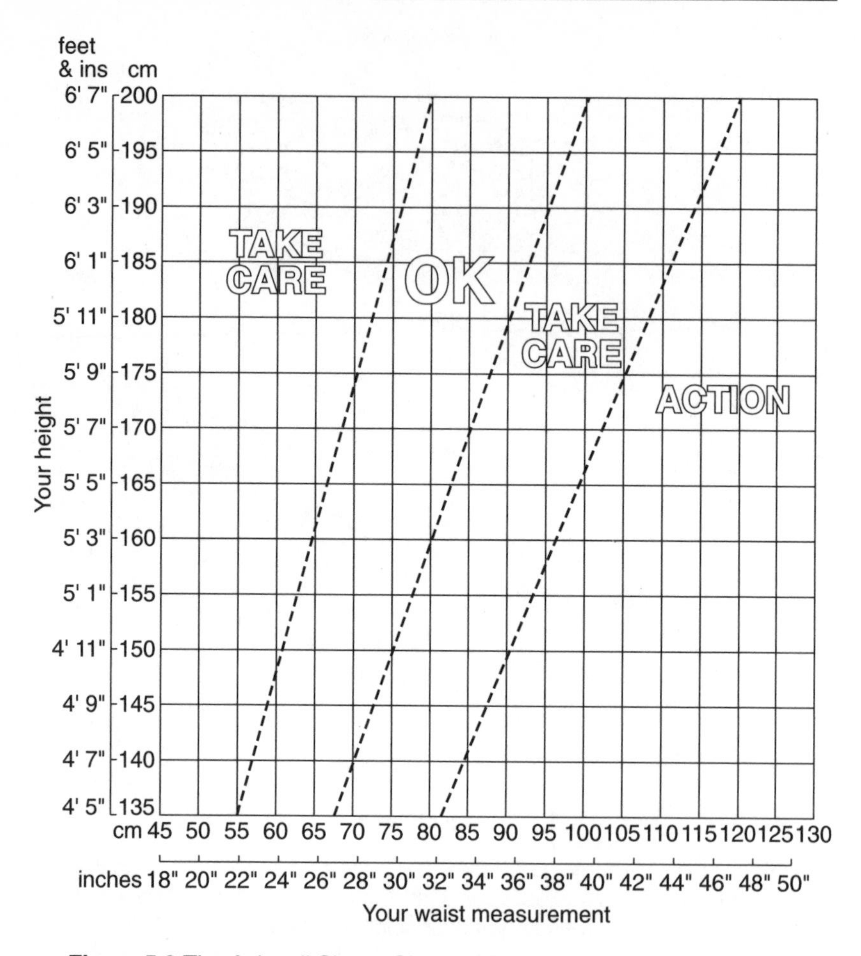

Figure 5.2 The Ashwell Shape Chart, which should help you to decide whether you have the correct (healthy) shape for your weight.
(© Dr Margaret Ashwell. Reproduced with permission)

based on grapefruit or cabbage soup, are more complicated than they need be; diets with special supplements may turn out to be expensive, and difficult to maintain when away from home. We suggest that you merely cut down on what you normally eat, rather than trying a completely different style of eating. Because fatty foods store energy in the most concentrated form, they should be cut in any calorie-controlled diet but, to avoid problems related to Type 2 diabetes, you should also drastically reduce carbohydrates such as refined sugar, confectionery, cakes, pasta, bread and starchy vegetables.

It is particularly important not to go on a crash diet, because a sudden loss of weight could bring on an acute attack of gouty arthritis. Aim to lose about half a kilo (about one pound) of weight per week; a gradual loss coupled with a change in eating habits should help you to maintain your new lower weight. As little as 30 minutes' brisk walking each day will also help to keep your weight down.

You may find it helpful to join a club that meets weekly for mutual encouragement, information . . . and regular weighing! Consult the telephone book or advertising in local newspapers for the nearest Weight Watchers or similar reputable organisation.

Drinking like a lord

Although I now understand that not only heavy drinkers get gout, how is alcohol connected with gouty attacks?

There are several long-term reasons why alcoholic beverages are particularly bad for people with gout.

- Beer is the greatest culprit: unfiltered real ales, 'Belgian'-style lagers, 'scrumpy' ciders and home-made wines contain yeast, which has a very high content of purine, and all beers and lagers also contain guanosine, a purine that is converted to uric acid in the gut.
- All alcoholic drinks and the mixers in cocktails (tonic, lemonade, cordials) are high in calories, so regular drinking may lead to overweight or even obesity.
- Particularly if food is not taken with alcohol, the consequent rise in lactic acid will increase the acidity of body fluids, and will also affect the ability of the kidneys to excrete uric acid.

- In alcoholics and heavy drinkers, gout is commonly caused by a combination of dehydration and not eating properly.

In the short term, some people report that their gouty attacks follow swiftly after an evening of unusually heavy drinking, whether with or without food. Two possible reasons are that, because alcohol is a diuretic, a 'binge' leads to dehydration (and a hangover headache), and the urine becomes more acid (see Chapter 3, ***Drugs to combat the pain and inflammation***). Either of these effects may bring on a gouty attack.

Does the effect of alcohol in gout mean that I have to go teetotal?

No, but if you drink more than the recommended healthy limits of 21 units per week for men or 14 units per week for women, you should be cutting back anyway, for the sake of your heart, liver and brain. A 'unit' is a surprisingly small amount – equivalent to a small glass of wine or half a pint of lager. Spirits, cocktails, Alcopops, fortified wines (e.g. port or sherry) and the more exotic beers all contain a higher concentration of alcohol, so you should be careful to drink even smaller amounts of these. Some people may find it less complicated to eliminate beer completely from their diet and their social life, but for others drinking less may be good enough. It is better to restrict alcohol to mealtimes rather than having several glasses of wine or beer without food.

I mostly drink wine rather than beer. Is white wine better for me than red?

White wine is just as likely to promote an attack of gouty arthritis as a red wine with similar alcohol content, if you drink a quantity without food and cause dehydration. The same goes for spirits. Nevertheless, some people report that red wines cause them particular problems, and it seems as if the only answer is to stop drinking them. It may be that red wines with a heavy deposit of tartrates (found at the bottom of the bottle) may bring on gouty attacks in susceptible people, so it is worth asking a wine merchant for some ideas of which wines to buy.

Historically, gout was associated with the drinking of port, which is usually red, and was not associated with drinking sherry, which is usually based on white wines. They are both fortified wines (alcohol content 19–22% compared with 10–14% in table wine). It should also be said that some people with gout drank huge quantities of port, as well as table wine, whereas sherry was perhaps considered to be an aperitif, served in smaller glasses. In the 'bad old days' port was often contaminated with lead that had leached out from the glass bottles or decanters, which were made of lead crystal. Port drinkers were thus being poisoned by the lead contaminant, which induced 'saturnine' gout, a secondary gout. Modern wine bottles are lead-free.

During my career in the restaurant trade, I drank wine every day – sometimes as much as two bottles in an evening – and I would say I have had a fair amount of vintage port. I did not have my first attack of gout until several years after I had retired, when my consumption of alcohol dropped quite drastically. I did have a friend who seemed to drink only Scotch, and he suffered terribly from gout from his forties.

When you were entertaining clients, you were presumably eating a meal and perhaps also drinking water. You were also probably more physically active during the day than you may be now you are retired. All of these factors can add up to keep gout away until later in life. Your friend's gout was a result of the diuretic and dehydrating effects of spirits on the system, which conspire to prevent the ready excretion of uric acid from the kidneys. We hope he now drinks a lot of water with his whisky!

Back to basics

Should I restrict the amount of purine-rich foods I eat, to prevent the formation of uric acid?

Yes, definitely! It is essential to know what foods are particularly high in purines (see Table 5.1, later in this chapter) so that you can control your own treatment. If you have been eating less food over all than previously, you will already have cut your intake of purines. If you are not overweight and do not have diabetes or high blood pressure, you do not need to cut calories but you should reduce the proportion of purine-rich food in your meals. Eat the same as the rest of the family but avoid the foods on the list that are very rich in purines. We have seen an attack of gout brought on within hours in susceptible people simply by feeding them pâté sandwiches or a large plate of seafood.

Remember that you should continue with allopurinol. Ask your doctor to test your plasma urate level and advise you when and if the dose of allopurinol can be reduced.

Children and young people with the metabolic disorders described in Chapter 6 (***Gout in young people***) already have a high level of purines in their body. So the advice to them about diet is as above, and they should take even more care to avoid any foods very rich in purines and to ensure that they drink plenty of fluids (mainly water) as well.

I'm trying to eat sensibly and avoid food rich in purines. Can you give me a list of all the foods I shouldn't eat?

Table 5.1 gives a summary of the figures obtained by analysing foodstuffs. Foods fall into the same category whether they are fresh, frozen, canned or dried, and in whatever way they are cooked, which makes it easier to keep track! The foods in the list are those that are easily available in supermarkets in the UK. You may eat some more exotic foods that we have not included, or you may hardly ever encounter some of the items that we mention – however, we hope the Table is helpful to most people.

Table 5.1 Purine content of foods

Group A: 0–50mg purine per 100g

fruits
vegetables – all except those in group B (runner/green/string beans, French beans, mange-tout and sugar-snap peas are all right)
cereals – all except those in group B (most bread and cakes, most breakfast cereals, biscuits, rice, barley, couscous, polenta and pasta are permitted in moderation)
dairy products (milk, cream, yoghurt, ice-cream, cheese, eggs – bearing in mind the high fat content of most dairy products)
fats, within reasonable calorie limits (butter, most cooking oils, lard, 'shortening', salad dressing, mayonnaise)
nuts – but not peanuts or cashew nuts, and preferably not salted nuts
olives
preserves (jam, marmalade, chutney, pickles) and sweets
beverages, including tea, coffee, soft drinks (but these may contain caffeine)

Group B: 50–150mg purine per 100g

poultry (chicken, duck, turkey, goose)
red meats (veal, beef, lamb, pork, bacon) and sausages
fish – except those in group C
oysters, mussels and most other shellfish, prawns, shrimps, scampi
wholegrain bread and pasta
wholegrain cereals (including oatmeal, brown rice and tahini)
lentils, soya beans, soya flour, bean curd, tofu, tempeh, miso, hummus, peas and beans, including chickpeas
peanuts, peanut butter, cashew nuts, ground nuts
brassicas (cauliflower, broccoli/calabrese, kale, Brussels sprouts, 'Chinese greens')
spinach, asparagus, avocado and mushrooms
Quorn

Group C: 150–1,000mg purine per 100g

wild or farmed game (pheasant, quail, grouse, rabbit/hare, venison)
organ meats (kidney, heart, sweetbreads, liver, pâté, terrine, liver sausage, foie gras)
extracts of meat and yeast (Bovril, Oxo, Marmite, Vegemite)
fish roe (cod roe, caviar, taramasalata)
scallops, herrings, mackerel, trout
crayfish, lobster
small fish eaten whole or processed (anchovies, sardines, sprats, whitebait, anchovy paste, Gentlemen's Relish, Thai fish sauce)

If you wish to take up a low-purine diet, you can eat anything from group A, and you should avoid all of group C. Foods from group B can be eaten in small quantities, and indeed they are required because many of them are significant sources of protein. You do not need to eliminate purines entirely from your diet.

The purine content of foods in the Table is calculated per 100 grams (a little less than 4 ounces), so you can 'trade' items to keep below about 200 milligrams of purine per day. A serving of 100 grams is equivalent to a small-to-moderate portion of meat, but it is a rather large portion of bread or pasta, and you are unlikely to eat more than a very small amount of some of the other foods. For example, a thin scraping of Marmite on toast would be all right if you don't eat beans or peas as well. Remember to keep portions small, and to restrict your intake of alcohol as far as possible.

The list of foods I should avoid or cut out completely leaves me with a really limited choice! I think the group letters, A B C, stand for 'always bread and cheese'. What on Earth can I eat apart from cheese sandwiches?

We like to think the letters mean 'Always Be Careful'. If you remember the types of food in each category, you will find that you quickly become accustomed to spotting group C items in prepared meals as they are presented to you or as you read a menu. Over all, our advice is to eat what you normally eat, but to avoid any of the purine-rich food listed in the Table or to take them infrequently in very small quantities. Many people get on very well without ever eating any of the group C foods.

Cheese, with its high proportion of animal fat, should not figure often in your meals, and the total calorie count should encourage the loss of weight if you are overweight, or you have diabetes or high blood pressure. Remember to eat only small portions of the group B foods and to drink plenty of water.

I suppose I'll learn – eventually – which foods belong in which group! Is there an easy way of working out whether a food is likely to be high in purines?

Yes, you can think about whether the food was obtained from a part of the animal or plant that was growing or metabolising rapidly (liver, kidney, cauliflower florets, asparagus tips), or that stored the capacity for growth (grain and seeds, fish eggs). Whole organisms that grow rapidly, such as yeast or fungi, will also contain a lot of nucleic acids and so will provide purines. Fats, white flour and fruit juices have been separated from the 'living' part of the food and so they are very low in purines. We do not need to eat purines because we make them in our body, so all that we take in as part of our diet is eventually excreted as uric acid.

I buy quite a lot of packaged foods and ready-meals. What should I look out for on the labels?

The ingredients listed first on the label will be the main components. Purines are not labelled but you should be able to see what proportion of a dish is meat or beans, for example. Ready-made dishes are often very high in salt, which can affect the filtration process in your kidneys. Remember to keep within the portion size recommended for one person.

How can I enjoy social occasions if I have to cut down on beer, calories and foods containing purines? I feel really depressed.

Our suggested changes to your lifestyle will help you to better general health as well as reducing the frequency or severity of gouty attacks. It sounds very hard at first, but the pain of gouty arthritis might help to remind you of the advantages of taking control of your diet!

Meals eaten on holiday or with friends often contain problem foods, and we all tend to over-eat on these occasions. However, you will usually be offered a choice of food items, and it should be possible to ask for something that won't be bad for you. There is nothing to prevent you from having one meat meal per day – just steer clear of feasts of seafood, pâté, lobster, beer, and wine without food. You can use the opportunity to try salads and exotic fruits. And of course, you don't have to eat everything that is put on your plate.

I love spinach, broccoli and asparagus – which are group B foods – but I've noticed that I seem to get an acute attack soon after eating them. Does this mean that I should cut them out completely?

These vegetables have quite a high level of purines in them, so if you eat a portion with some meat, you may produce more uric acid than your kidneys can cope with. Perhaps you could eat them as part of a salad or a stir-fry meal with little or no meat, or just cut down on the portion size of these vegetables if you are having them with the Sunday lunch.

Some foods that trigger my attacks (strawberries and citrus fruit) are not on the 'high-purine' list. Do you think they could be hindering the excretion of uric acid from other foods? If so, has any research been done into foods that have an opposite, beneficial effect – behaving like the urate-lowering drugs?

Several people have reported 'trigger' foods that are not high in purines, and, having proved the point to their own satisfaction, they just avoid eating these foods. We suspect that sodium citrate (in citrus fruit) or calcium oxalate (in tomatoes and strawberries) may have some effect on how much uric acid can dissolve in body fluids, but we have no direct evidence for this. Some people with gout report that an attack may be brought on by eating nuts; both nuts and liver contain a high concentration of niacin (vitamin B_3), which may slow down the excretion of urate into the urine.

We can't find any research that has been done specifically into low-purine foods that can help people with gout. A nutritionist has suggested to us that phyto-oestrogens – molecules resembling female sex hormones – found in foods such as soya, may help in the excretion of uric acid, although there is no hard evidence for this. Breads made with soya flour have recently featured in popular medicine articles as an alternative to hormone replacement therapy for women; because depletion of the female hormones is thought to be the first step towards gout in older women, a few slices of the bread may be a useful addition to your diet. Such 'HRT' breads may be available in your local health food shop, or in larger supermarkets. Bear in mind, though, that this bread will fall into group B in Table 5.1, because of the soya flour. You may like to try some of recipes that embrace this approach – look out for the book *Natural Alternatives to HRT Cookbook* in your library or bookshop (details in Appendix 2, ***Useful publications***).

A friend has told me that cherries help in the excretion of uric acid. How can I test that idea?

This is a new one to us! It may be a variation on the uricosuric effect of high doses of vitamin C, which we have already described in Chapter 3 (***Drugs to combat the pain and inflammation***). We wouldn't recommend that you give up your prescription and rely entirely on cherries but you could test their effect if you sometimes get gouty arthritis. Without altering other aspects of your diet or drug regimen, see if the attacks are less frequent or less painful when you eat cherries regularly (two or three times per week?) over a period of a few weeks or months. The season for fresh cherries is very short, so you'll have to find a source for tinned, frozen or dried cherries or the juice.

A medical website on the internet says that people with gout should cut down on the amount of protein in their diet. Does this help to stop the uric acid crystals from forming?

Protein is the third major component of our diet, along with carbohydrate and fat. It is essential to eat some protein every day, though perhaps not as much as Westerners often do. Proteins are biochemically completely distinct from the nucleic acids that release purines when they are digested. Nevertheless, some foods that are rich in protein are also rich in purines – organ meat (e.g. kidney, liver), shellfish, beans – so the website advice is broadly correct, with some important exceptions. For example, cheese and yoghurt are rich in protein but low in purines, while some vegetables are high in purines without being a particularly good source of protein. Eliminating meat (especially game and organ meats) from your diet will reduce both purines and protein but you must include other proteins in your diet.

Dr Patrick Dessein, at the Baragwanath Hospital in Soweto, South Africa, has devised an eating plan that helped to reduce the frequency and severity of gouty attacks in men who were overweight or obese but not heavy drinkers. His research suggests that it is more important to reduce the overall amount of food – to about 1,600 calories per day for a man – rather than cutting the proportion of protein. Ideally, each meal consists of protein + carbohydrate + fats, with an overall calorie distribution of 30 per cent, 40 per cent, 30 per cent respectively. Bear in mind that each gram of fat contains about twice as many calories as a gram of carbohydrate. His regimen did not eliminate foods from group B (as listed in Table 5.1), but group C foods were not eaten. This diet therefore combines restriction of calories and purines. The men in the study were not treated with urate-lowering drugs at the time, so they did continue to have gouty attacks, although less severely than before.

I'm not overweight although I have to eat out frequently with business clients. I keep myself fit with running and weight training. I always choose dishes that are low in calories and fat, and I drink only one glass of wine with the meal. Nevertheless, at the age of 52, I have been diagnosed with primary gout. How can this be?

The slight decline in the removal of uric acid by the kidney happens naturally even to fit men whose weight is normal – it is not a punishment for a bad life! You are likely to be one of the small number of people with a genetic predisposition to gout. Your weight is normal, but it is possible that your diet includes several foods that are high in purines – they occur frequently on restaurant menus. Organ meats (pâté, liver, kidney) or game, seafood, mushrooms, avocado, asparagus and broccoli may seem innocuous in terms of calories but they can provide significant amounts of purines.

When you are running or training at the gym, be sure to drink enough water or 'isotonic sports drink' (which, unlike more concentrated fruit drinks, tends not to promote dehydration by acting as a diuretic) to compensate for loss of fluid through perspiration. Weigh yourself before and after exercise, and drink about 1.5 litres for every kilogram lost. You might consider taking up cycling or swimming instead of running, to relieve the pressure on your feet, and beware of explosive effort in, for example, squash or football.

I find watching what I eat and drink very frustrating. Why do I still have to do this now that I'm taking these drugs?

You will have been given drugs to control the high levels of uric acid that continue to accumulate in your blood. This is a long-term (lifetime) therapy – few people can succeed with diet alone. Allopurinol will help to slow down the rate at which uric acid builds up in your blood. Uricosuric drugs will help to eliminate uric acid when it reaches your kidneys. The fact still remains, however, that high-purine foods will raise urate levels in your blood so that eventually crystals will form. It makes sense to think about your intake of meat, seafood and alcohol – especially beer.

If you have been prescribed a very low dose of allopurinol, or you take tablets on alternate days, it could indicate that your kidneys are not working very efficiently, and therefore your doctor will be very glad if you can help by restricting your intake of beer and purine-rich foods. The doctor will be hoping that you can control the amount of purine in your diet so that the dose of allopurinol need not be raised for a while. For people with the metabolic gout described in Chapter 6 (***Gout in young people***), it is generally not wise to have a dose of more than 300mg allopurinol per day because of the danger of accumulating too much xanthine in the kidneys.

Mealtimes

My husband is overweight because he has always enjoyed good food and drink, and now he has gout. Can I protect my teenage sons from getting this condition in the future?

A substantial minority of men have inherited the tendency (predisposition) to gout, so you are right to be concerned about your sons, though the problem should only occur in their middle age. You can certainly provide more salads and fruit, and perhaps pasta dishes or stir-fries that contain less meat and fewer group B or C foods in your meals at home – which will help your husband – and hope that you are training the boys to think carefully about their diet in general so that they eat healthily and do not become overweight. When they are out with their friends they may binge on food as well as beer, and there's not a lot you can do about that except warn them of the danger of drinking beer without having food. If they leave home to go to college, they will have to cook some meals themselves, and you can help by giving them some ideas for low-fat, low-purine meals that are quick and economical. We list a few recipe books in Appendix 2 (***Useful publications***).

My sister feeds vegetarian food to her family, so this should help her husband's gout, shouldn't it?

It is certainly a good start because meat, fish and poultry are the major sources of purines in the diet, and they are presumably missing from your sister's meals. However, without good nutritional advice, it is possible to eat a 'bad' vegetarian diet – high in cheese, eggs, bread – unless you get vegetable proteins from nuts, beans and cereals. Pulses (peas, beans and lentils) are a significant source of protein but note that these foods are in group B – fairly good sources of purines, too. Soya flour, bean curd, tofu and Quorn are also in this group. These products are very useful as substitutes for a meat meal. Incidentally, the well-known 'wind' problem that affects many vegetarians may be helped by charcoal tablets; these absorb the methane released from beans and cabbage.

Has your sister seen anything like the list of food groups shown in Table 5.1? If not, she might be grateful for a copy of the Table to help her plan meals that will be all right for her husband.

Vegetarians, especially those who don't eat any animal products such as eggs and cheese, will need to take a supplement containing vitamin B_{12}.

If your brother-in-law eats non-vegetarian meals with colleagues at work, he should have only small portions of meat and of other foods that fall into group B in our list.

Do you have any ideas for a good cookery book with tasty recipes that can be used to help gout?

We can't find a book written specifically with low-purine foods in mind, apart from two books published in the USA and available through the internet (www.gout-haters.com). Sample recipes shown might appeal more to the US market than to UK readers.

If you are interested in preparing food from fresh ingredients, using good nutritional principles, you will want books containing a wide range of recipes that can be enjoyed by the whole family and guests. You can compile your own collection of favourites from several books. Look in your local library for books on food and health to 'try before you buy'. We can recommend the titles listed in Appendix 2 (***Useful publications***), but there are undoubtedly more.

You will need to make a note to avoid recipes that contain ingredients falling in Group C of Table 5.1, because the advice to cut purines does not correspond to cutting calories or any of the major components of food (protein, fat and carbohydrate).

I seem to have attacks when I have had a busy day without time to stop for lunch or a tea break. Does this make sense?

The regular rhythm by which uric acid is excreted may have been put out of kilter by your missing lunch, especially if you compensate by eating more in the evening. You may also have drunk less fluid than needed to flush out the urate from your evening meal, hence a gouty attack the next morning.

Is it best to keep to regular mealtimes or to eat several small meals through the day?

It seems more sensible to eat a larger meal at lunchtime so that there is time for your body to excrete uric acid during the day. This is not usually possible if you are out at work, so whatever arrangement you have should be maintained at weekends. Don't 'skip' meals: try to keep to a regular routine that fits in with other members of the family.

You will also need to drink at least two litres of fluid, spread over the day and evening. Getting up at night to pass urine is a small inconvenience compared with a gouty attack.

Why do diet sheets always recommend huge quantities of water?

You will have been told to drink enough to make you pass at least two litres of urine per day. A two-litre bottle is equivalent to six normal-sized cans of cola or six to eight mugs of hot drinks. You would not be wise to drink two litres of cola or brewed coffee – they have a higher caffeine content than recommended for general health and they may slow the excretion of uric acid from your kidneys. Diet sheets recommend water rather than other drinks because water does not contribute calories, unlike milk (in the form of fat) or fruit juice (in the form of sugar). If you usually have sugar in tea or coffee, you will cut calories by dropping some of those drinks in exchange for water or another drink. Because alcoholic drinks are discouraged for the reasons given earlier in this chapter, you wouldn't think of beer or wine as a significant source of fluid. You could try infusions, or hot drinks, made with herbs or flowers. Flavoured teas, in which a fruit flavouring is added to India or China tea, still contain caffeine, and guarana, which is a herbal equivalent to caffeine, should be avoided. Some naturally caffeine-free teas and decaffeinated coffee can be found in most supermarkets and health food shops.

I am trying to organise the food for my daughter's wedding reception, and I have just learned that the groom's father and uncle have gout. Do you have any suggestions?

You could plan a buffet, or offer a choice of main courses for a sit-down meal, bearing in mind the high-purine foods listed in Table 5.1. As some of the guests may be vegetarians, or have diabetes, lactose intolerance or an allergy to nuts, you cannot provide a special menu for each person. However, you can ask the caterers to bear in mind those who have different requirements, and to offer a choice of dishes.

Drinking before the main meal is a potential problem for everybody at a convivial occasion like this, and especially for people with gout, so provide plenty of festive alternatives such as sparkling mineral water, lemonade and fruit juices.

Give your daughter a copy of this book and a good recipe book (see Appendix 2, ***Useful publications***), so she can help her new husband, who may be at risk.

My wife and I enjoy trying foreign foods on holiday. What can we do to avoid problems?

Take a phrase book with a good 'restaurant' section so that you can understand the menu, or write your own list of 'forbidden' foods in the appropriate language. All national cuisines have a staple food that is based on carbohydrate, so you should not go hungry even if you find you have to eat rice, potatoes or bread because you ordered liver casserole by mistake. Be careful to eat according to your usual diet and to drink enough fluid while you are travelling. You could take a large bottle of mineral water on the journey, especially if travelling by air. When on holiday, eat regularly – bread and fruit, if nothing else! Avoid too much exercise in the heat, because of the danger of dehydration. Check that your travel insurance covers likely emergencies, and carry a small supply of emergency drugs (e.g. colchicine or an NSAID) in case you have a gouty attack while you are away.

If my diet is restricted according to this plan for avoiding purine-rich foods, should I take a vitamin supplement?

Is your diet really restricted? You may be eating less than previously but, if you eat a range of different foods, you should be getting enough vitamins and minerals. It's true that some minerals may be deficient in some people but a balanced diet should usually contain all the tiny traces that are needed.

The one-pill-a-day vitamin supplements sold in pharmacies usually contain about the right daily level of vitamins, and, if you must, these are the ones to buy. The ingredients, and their relationship to the recommended daily amount (RDA), should always be shown on the packaging or label. Look for those giving between 80 and 100 per cent of the RDA. Some 'specialist' supplements, for example mixtures advertised for perking up the stressed office worker, contain nine or ten times the RDA for several vitamins. An extra-high dose of vitamins can give you too much of the chemicals, such as niacin (vitamin B_3), riboflavin (vitamin B_2) and nicotinic acid, that reduce the ability of the kidneys to excrete uric acid, so you should avoid them. Vitamin tablets based on brewers' yeast, and formulations of blue–green algae (*Spirulina*), should also be avoided because of their high purine content.

Vitamin C tablets sold for the prevention of the common cold suggest a dose, spread over the day, of up to 3 grams, which is 50 times the RDA for this vitamin (60 milligrams). The uricosuric effect of such high doses can be beneficial (but may be complicated by stomach upsets) and you should tell your doctor if you are taking other uricosuric drugs. The increased excretion of uric acid could cause confusion if your doctor asks for a measurement of your plasma urate levels.

Sometimes I feel a bit low so I have been drinking Red Bull, which is advertised as a pick-me-up or 'energy' drink. Does this contain anything that I shouldn't be taking?

It does contain at least as much caffeine as a cup of strong coffee. The same applies to ProPlus tablets (caffeine citrate), which many students take when studying or writing essays late at night. There isn't really an alternative, if you are determined not to go to bed – just be aware of what you are taking.

6

Gout in young people

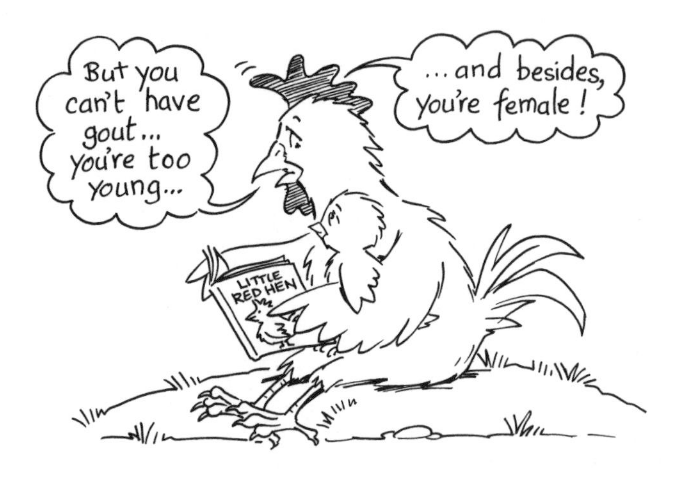

Children of either sex and women and men in their 20s do not normally develop gout, because they excrete uric acid more efficiently than middle-aged and older men. Consequently, if they develop arthritis-like symptoms suddenly, or a tophus is found, it may take some time for gout to be even considered. Gout in all these cases is generally a side-effect of an underlying disease. So it is vital that parents as well as doctors recognise that gout in women or young men is *always unusual* and a specialist centre must be contacted to find the cause. Other young people in the same family may also be affected although not yet showing symptoms. Treatment, as well as advice, will differ from that given for classic 'primary' gout.

These rare disorders (less than 5 per cent of all cases of gout) either are the result of a disturbance in the 'production line' – the uncontrolled production of purines normally recycled by the body – or arise because much less uric acid is being excreted by the kidneys. Such conditions lead to excessively high levels of urate or uric acid in the blood and sometimes in the urine, and can be damaging to the kidneys as well, especially in situations that lead to dehydration (infections, vomiting, diarrhoea, etc.). Diet is still important in the face of the massive overload of the body's system, because high-purine foods can raise blood levels of urate in an already saturated system, and thereby trigger a gouty attack. Other symptoms may be seen, including distressing cerebral palsy in some, or rapidly progressive kidney disease (if untreated) in others – sometimes both – but these vary considerably. Allopurinol can help some of the gout symptoms but must be used with great care.

The important and urgent requirement is to obtain a correct diagnosis so that the gout can be treated, and other family members can be tested so that appropriate advice can be given swiftly.

Familial juvenile hyperuricaemic nephropathy

Familial juvenile hyperuricaemic nephropathy (FJHN) – 'familial juvenile gout' for short – is a disorder in which young people are unable to excrete uric acid as efficiently as expected for their age. This leads to a raised level of uric acid in young men or women, or in children of either sex; the hyperuricaemia is even higher than in the typical middle-aged gouty man. An attack of gout in such a young person has often drawn attention to a family previously considered to have a mysterious 'familial renal disease' stretching over several generations. If the disorder is unrecognised and untreated – or recognised but not treated sufficiently early with allopurinol – it can result in a rapid decline in the efficiency of the kidneys, needing dialysis and then transplantation at an early age.

My twin sister developed gout in her big toe when she was 9 and was found to have damaged kidneys. I was investigated too and found to have a very high uric acid but no gout. My mother and two aunts died of kidney disease in their 30s. Both my sister and I were put onto allopurinol, which has helped me but my sister died recently at 38. Why was there a difference in outcome?

The outlook (prognosis) with allopurinol is good, but only if you are treated when your kidneys still have at least half their ability to excrete uric acid. Allopurinol slows down further damage to the kidneys.

It is likely that you began treatment early enough but, because your sister's kidneys were already working inefficiently, it was too late for allopurinol to be as effective. Your mother and aunts had the condition before allopurinol was introduced, and presumably already had damaged kidneys. Remember that you must take your allopurinol daily, effectively for the rest of your life.

Will my FJHN be passed on to all my children?

This is a 'dominant inherited disorder', meaning that, theoretically, you can pass this on to half your children whether they are boys or girls. This can be seen in the imaginary family tree in Figure 6.1. The black shapes are people with FJHN; circles are female, squares are male. You can see that half of the people in the middle generation have the disorder and that half of the children of an affected person have FJHN, too. However, note that a person who does not have FJHN herself does not have the gene to pass on to her children. If we imagine that you are an affected person in the middle of the diagram, we can predict that statistically half your children will be affected, although an element of chance operates. Thus, you may find that all your children are free of the condition and it should not recur in subsequent generations in the family, or alternatively that all of them have unfortunately inherited the faulty gene.

FJHN can be detected by finding a very high urate value (i.e. above the normal values for people of the same age and sex) in

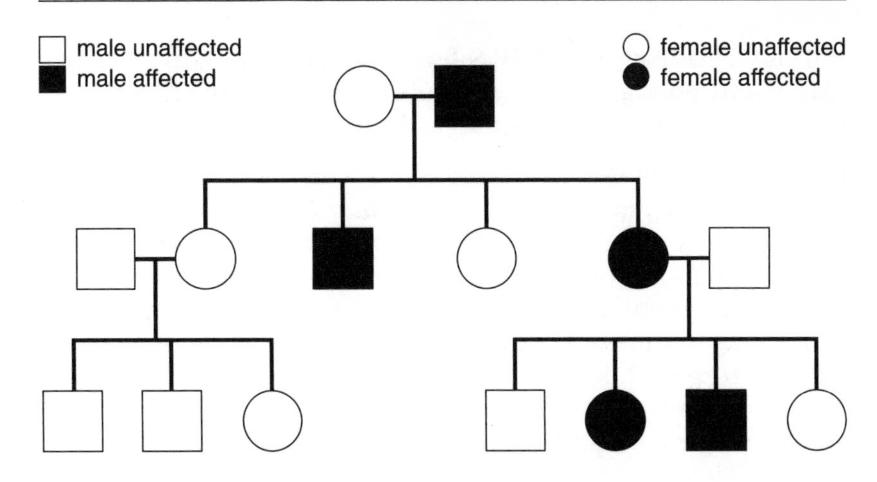

Figure 6.1 An idealised example of a family tree of people affected by FJHN. You can see that half of the people in the middle generation have the disorder (the black shapes) and that half of the children of an affected person have FJHN, too.

the blood *and* much less uric acid in the urine compared with values for healthy children on a low-purine diet. The children who are not affected (those with normal values of plasma urate and urine uric acid) have no 'bad' gene to pass on to the next generation.

Do I understand that this 'juvenile gout' is a childhood form of the classic gout that you have described in middle-aged men?

No, not really. Middle-aged people with primary gout who are treated with allopurinol to control their urate levels generally have normally functioning kidneys for their age today. However, you are correct to assume that FJHN reflects a problem in the kidneys, preventing the excretion of uric acid derived from food and drink.

Will my children with FJHN have to expect frequent acute attacks of podagra, damaged joints and perhaps also tophus formation in other sites in the body?

Gout is a rare but useful 'marker' of this condition, drawing attention to one of the aspects of a familial disease that may have seemed to be connected only with the kidneys. However, the serious symptoms of gout that you mention may occur if affected youngsters do not take their allopurinol regularly, or if they keep consuming purine-rich foods and beverages. It is sometimes difficult to get children and teenagers to comply with regular drugs and a restricted diet, but you should be frank with them about the dire consequences if they do not toe the line!

Two of my children have FJHN. Will they get kidney stones or develop kidney failure as a result?

Uric acid kidney stones are not a feature of FJHN. If this disorder is diagnosed and treated with allopurinol early enough – *and they take their drug daily* – your children's kidneys should remain healthy. They should be monitored, however, to ensure that the allopurinol dose is correct (see also the next question and answer).

My 5-year-old son has no symptoms so far but he has been diagnosed with the family disorder of gout and kidney disease. My doctor is reluctant to prescribe the allopurinol that we all take daily, because it will be for life. What should I do?

We know of a teenager who had normal kidneys when first diagnosed with FJHN but was not given allopurinol. In seven years, half of the ability to excrete uric acid had been lost, but his kidney function has now stabilised on allopurinol, and of course the tendency to gout is also diminished.

You should ask your doctor to refer your son to your local paediatric nephrologist (children's kidney specialist) or to the renal unit of the regional hospital. They will help to decide on a suitable dose of allopurinol, which has a vital role in reducing levels of uric acid. Your doctor will monitor urate levels in your son's blood to check this. Your son should also eat a low-purine diet (see Chapter 5, ***Food and drink***).

The earlier you can train your son to take his tablets daily, the better it will be. If he ever objects to this routine, remind him that many people have no problems in voluntarily taking vitamin tablets – or jelly beans – daily.

My daughter feels very upset to have gout at such a young age, and in fact as a family we are all rather dismayed by the diagnosis of FJHN. Can you put me in touch with any self-help groups?

Yes. PUMPA (the Purine Metabolic Patients' Association) has a patient contact member who will put families in touch with one another if they so wish. Other organisations help families with a range of disabilities and problems. Their contact details are given in Appendix 1, ***Useful addresses***.

Other metabolic disorders associated with high uric acid levels and gout

Both *Lesch–Nyhan disease* (LND) and *phosphoribosylpyrophosphate synthetase* super-activity (PRPS) are rare X-linked disorders, affecting mostly boys. This is because one of the two sex-determining, or X, chromosomes in the mother's cells has a faulty gene that can be carried into half of her children. Daughters will not usually develop the condition because their second X chromosome (from their father) will usually have a gene for a normal enzyme. However, half of the girls will be 'carriers' like their mother – they will be able to pass the faulty gene on to their children even though they are not themselves affected by it. Half of the sons will have the faulty X chromosome, and, because the Y chromosome in male cells does not carry a 'good' copy of the relevant gene, these sons will be affected by the disorder. See

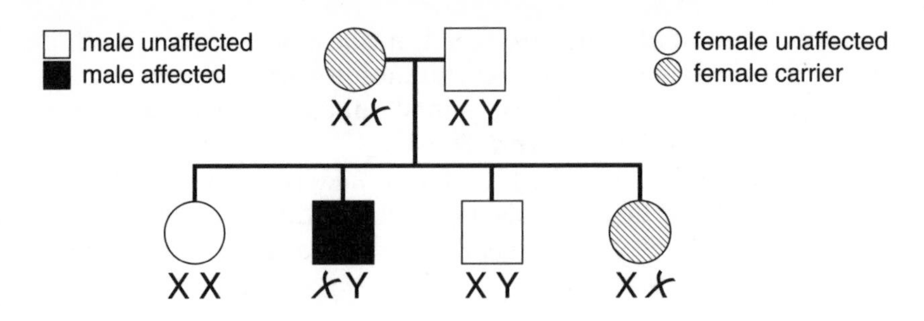

Figure 6.2 This simplified family tree shows that the children of a mother carrying the faulty X chromosome (shown as a bent X) are statistically likely to include an affected son (black square) and a daughter who also carries the faulty X chromosome (shaded circle). Because this daughter also has a normal X chromosome from her father, she is not affected by the condition: she is a 'carrier'.

Figure 6.2 for an example of the family tree of children of a woman who is a carrier.

In LND an enzyme with a dreadful name – hypoxanthine guanine phosphoribosyltransferase (HPRT) – cannot recycle the purines from the daily wear and tear in your body. Thus the mechanism that normally sends a 'Stop – enough!' message to the production line is missing, and more purines are made uncontrollably. When the enzyme is completely absent, severe cerebral palsy (seen as involuntary self-injury, and inability to walk or talk in the first years of life) and acute kidney failure, sometimes with gout, happen in some children. It has been known for some children to have been institutionalised for 'cerebral palsy of unknown cause', only to be diagnosed with HPRT deficiency after puberty, when the first gout symptoms became apparent.

Such symptoms are less severe in *Kelley–Seegmiller syndrome* (KSS) and the milder LND variants, when the HPRT enzyme is only partly deficient or defective. But here, too, babies as well as teenagers can experience acute renal failure, caused by high concentrations of uric acid in their kidneys, following dehydration or a fever. Such variants generally show up as gout only after puberty, because children clear their uric acid better; most start having symptoms in their 20s. The LND variants also have mild degrees of movement disability – walking with an uncontrolled gait or swaying like a Greek dancer (choreo-athetosis).

The same over-production of uric acid happens when the enzyme PRPS, which controls the start of the production line, fails to respond to 'Stop – enough!' signals, and continues to produce large quantities of purines. Gross over-production of uric acid leads to very high levels of uric acid in the person's blood *and* urine. Gout, kidney stones or acute renal failure can result in children or adults. In this disorder, unlike with LND, the carrier mother may develop gout.

Incidence and diagnosis

What is the chance of my having a child with one of these X-linked disorders, and what is the prognosis for the child in either case?

PRPS is very rare indeed. Only one family has been found so far in the UK. Sadly, none of the three affected sons lived beyond the age of 8 years. About 40 families have been reported world-wide. The defect that causes LND or KSS is more common: about five new cases are diagnosed in the UK annually, about one-third being a new gene defect not previously seen in the family. The prognosis with LND has improved immensely since the disorder was first described. It will depend on how early the condition is diagnosed, and will require considerable input from family and carers. Much can be achieved by using aids to develop speech and walking and to control self-injury (e.g. bandages or splints on the hands and arms, specially constructed chairs with head restraints, and plastic tooth guards), plus adequate control of uric acid levels.

I am a 30-year-old woman and have gout. My two sons could not walk or talk, and they persistently had orange–red crystals on their nappies. The boys were tested for LND but found to have normal HPRT enzyme activity, so my GP was unable to help in the diagnosis. More recently, further samples from my sons and also from me were sent away to be tested at a specialist unit, which reported PRPS super-activity. What is this disorder and why do I have gout?

The crystals on the nappies were uric acid and your sons were found to have this very rare disorder (described earlier), in which the uric acid 'production line' is deaf to all 'Stop' messages. Gout in young women is very unusual, too. It does occur in FJHN (see earlier) but is not found in mothers of children with LND or KSS. Even though these women are carriers of the faulty gene, they are able to cope with moderate depletion of the HPRT activity. However, in the case of PRPS, mothers (and sisters with the faulty X chromosome) do have high levels of uric acid in the blood, and some will develop gout.

Because the disorder is so rare, you may be the only person with PRPS that your GP will see in his or her whole career, but the specialist unit will be more familiar with PRPS and the outlook for the future.

I am my wife's second husband, and we plan a new family in addition to her other children, one of whom has LND. What are the chances of her having another child with the same X-linked disorder?

The statistics are just the same as in her first marriage, because the defective gene is on an X chromosome carried in all her cells (see Figure 6.2). Half of your prospective daughters will be carriers and half the boys will be affected.

So, girls are never affected by LND, KSS or PRPS because the gene is on one X chromosome and they have another as a back-up?

Girls would usually expect to inherit a normal gene on the X chromosome from their father's sperm. Although girls with one faulty X chromosome are carriers of the defect, they should continue to be healthy because the good gene, and not the faulty gene, is used to make the HPRT enzyme in girls and women. However, once in a while a girl will develop symptoms of LND or KSS, but this is very uncommon, and may only be recognised when a brother with the same symptoms receives a correct diagnosis.

In the case of PRPS the mutation in the gene causes an overactivity, not a loss, of a normal enzyme. As a result, women and girls with one faulty gene for PRPS do have an excess of urate and they can get gout.

My 6-year-old son was rushed to hospital with acute renal failure after being given ampicillin for an infection. This was diagnosed as acute tubular blockage caused by uric acid. He recovered after dialysis and is now growing normally. Is he likely to have this problem again?

Tests in a specialist laboratory may find that he has inherited KSS. This is similar to LND but does not include cerebral palsy. Your son's body produces high levels of uric acid but his cells contain enough HPRT enzyme to escape the other problems of LND. However, some LND variants do exist, causing much milder disorders of movement, so that boys' symptoms are intermediate between LND and KSS. Only a specialist unit can tell the difference, from a blood and urine test. Your son will need allopurinol, but in a low dose to prevent kidney damage from the formation of xanthine stones.

The blockage in the kidneys occurred when the concentrations of uric acid rose rapidly above its solubility in his urine and crystals were deposited, blocking the kidney tubules. This happened because he probably developed diarrhoea, which, with the high temperature during his infection, made him dehydrated. The ampicillin will have stopped his kidneys reabsorbing uric acid, leading to an even higher level of uric acid in the already 'super-saturated' urine. It is important to ensure that your son drinks plenty of water when his temperature rises, and that he is not given ampicillin again if he has a bacterial infection.

My daughter has a boy with LND. She is frightened to get pregnant again in case her second child also has it.

Your daughter must be a carrier if she has already had an affected child. She can ask to be referred for genetic counselling so that she can explore her options. If she becomes pregnant again, she should be referred to her obstetrician for prenatal diagnosis early in the pregnancy. If the baby is male, his cells will carry only one X chromosome, and there is a 50 per cent chance that he will have the disorder (this also applies for PRPS). She and her partner might then wish to consider the options available, which can include terminating the pregnancy. Further analyses will be done to compare the genes in the unborn baby with the faulty gene present in your daughter's cells, as well as assaying the enzyme activity in the cells of the baby. If the baby is female, she will have a 50 per cent chance of inheriting the faulty gene on an X chromosome, but will generally be healthy.

Do you have other daughters? If the mutation is known, the DNA from all the girls in the family can be tested to see if they, too, are carriers.

My grandson was admitted to intensive care, aged one month, in acute renal failure. No one knew what had caused this and he had many tests. A doctor specialising in kidney problems in adults was called in and she noted that the baby had a very swollen finger (see Figure 6.3) – as in adults with gout – and said he should be tested for purine enzymes. It seems he has a disorder known as LND. Why did this happen, since it doesn't run in the family?

The diagnosis of an inherited disorder can be surprising, as X-linked disorders can be passed 'silently' from mother to

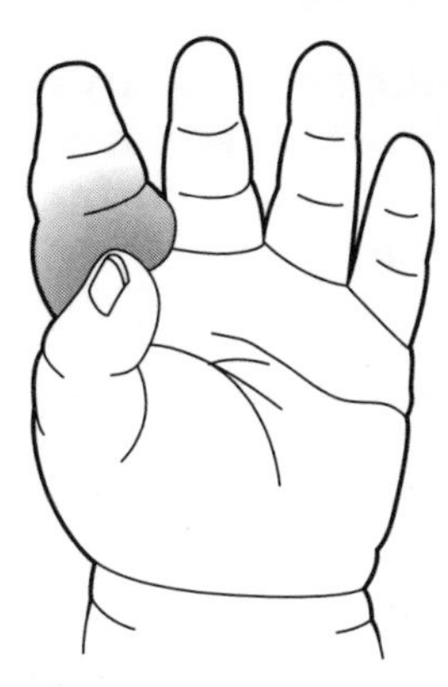

Figure 6.3 A baby's hand with a swollen finger, indicating the likelihood of LND.

daughter through several generations (see Figure 6.2). The faulty gene is usually detected only when carrying out tests in a boy who suffers from the lack of normal enzyme activity, as in the case of your grandson. It is also possible that a new mutation occurred in the egg that provided half your grandson's DNA.

The specialist laboratory was able to show that your grandson had inherited *complete* HPRT deficiency – LND – and thus his body was vastly over-producing uric acid. Because children excrete their uric acid very well, LND patients often have a normal level in blood plasma. Acute renal failure can develop in children with LND because their urine is saturated with uric acid. The urine is more acid than blood, causing excessive amounts of uric acid itself to be deposited as crystals in the kidney tubules, because he is producing and excreting too much. Prolonged formation of the crystals may eventually cause permanent kidney damage.

Your grandson should now be taking allopurinol as long-term therapy for the kidneys, but in a tiny dose to prevent kidney damage from the formation of xanthine stones. He should also be taking potassium citrate to make his urine more alkaline and to help the uric acid to stay in solution rather than forming crystals.

My first son has developed normally (he is now 8 years old) but his brother was diagnosed with LND at 18 months. Should we be looking out for symptoms of gout or renal failure in our older boy?

The diagnosis of LND in the baby will have been made on the basis of a complete lack of the HPRT gene normally found on the X chromosome, as we described earlier in this section. The absence of symptoms in the older brother suggests that he is OK and has the 'good' X chromosome from his mother and so the HPRT activity is normal. Nevertheless, he should be tested to confirm that he has a normal enzyme, in which case he will develop normally and will not pass on the condition to his own children.

My nephew was admitted to a care home when young, for 'cerebral palsy of unknown cause'. LND was ruled out because he had a normal blood urate measurement for his age, and he has not shown any sign of self-injuring behaviour. Now a teenager, he has suddenly developed gout. What is wrong?

Cerebral palsy has many causes, but the gout symptoms must have arisen from high concentrations of urate in his blood, which suggests that severe HPRT deficiency is the correct diagnosis. He does not have all the symptoms of LND because his body probably has some enzyme activity, which protects him from the more serious developmental problems that occur when there is a complete lack of the enzyme. When he was younger, his kidneys were excreting uric acid so efficiently that the plasma urate levels were in the normal range for children (lower than in adults). Thorough testing includes careful measurement of uric acid in the urine (gentle warming in the laboratory will re-dissolve any crystals that have formed during its collection) as well as measurement of the HPRT enzyme in a blood sample. Allopurinol must be prescribed, but with care to prevent kidney damage from the formation of xanthine stones rather than uric acid.

My teenage son was recently diagnosed with KSS. His elder sister has worked out that she may also have the faulty gene, so naturally she is concerned about having children herself. How can we find out if she is a carrier, and what about any children my son might have?

Your daughter has two X chromosomes, one from each parent. Even if she has a faulty HPRT gene on the X chromosome from her mother, her blood will probably *not* contain more uric acid than normal, because all of her cells have one copy of the normal HPRT gene and thus will contain the enzyme. We can only tell definitely if she is a carrier by getting a DNA sample from her blood and actually studying the structure of the HPRT gene in her DNA to see if it contains the same faulty region as in her brother. This can be done at a specialist centre.

If your daughter is found to be a carrier (as shown in Figure 6.2), she can ask for prenatal testing when she becomes pregnant; it is likely that half of her sons will be affected and half of her daughters will be carriers.

Because your son appears to be getting on well, it seems that KSS will not affect his ability to marry and to father children himself. In this case, as shown in Figure 6.4, we can be confident that

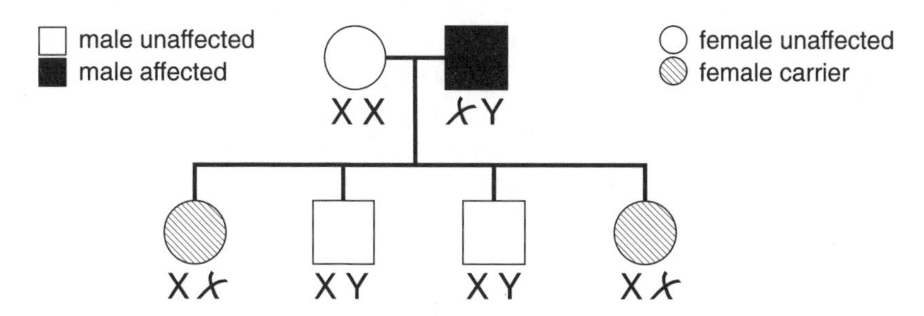

Figure 6.4 An idealised family tree of descendants from a male affected by one of several known X-linked disorders, such as KSS. It shows that, in this case, none of the sons will be affected by the condition because they will inherit the Y chromosome from their father, but all of the daughters will inherit the faulty X chromosome (shown as a bent X) and thus will be carriers.

none of his sons will inherit the condition (because they will inherit the Y chromosome from him), but all of his daughters will be carriers because they will have the faulty X chromosome.

Our baby son has had some fits and the doctors don't know what has caused them. He is small for his age and not developing normally. I've noticed that his nappies smell funny and there are orange–red bits where the urine has soaked in.

The orange crystals on the nappies suggest that his urine contains a very high concentration of some insoluble component. Ask your GP to have your son's blood tested for enzymes and nucleotides, and the urine tested for uric acid. It is possible that he has inherited a genetic disorder from his mother (either HPRT deficiency or PRPS, as described earlier in this chapter) and as a result his body makes very high levels of uric acid.

The alternative cause of high plasma urate in children, FJHN, does not lead to crystals on the nappies because these children under-excrete uric acid, and there is no associated cerebral palsy or problems with walking.

We are familiar with two other genetic purine disorders that can be recognised first by the mother noting crystals on the nappies. They are called *2,8-dihydroxyadenine lithiasis* and *xanthine lithiasis*. Neither disorder leads to any problems in the nervous system and each is treatable if recognised. Both disorders, if unrecognised and untreated, may eventually lead to the need for kidney dialysis and transplantation, so it is vital to distinguish these crystals from uric acid by special testing. These disorders are not connected with gout, but severe renal disease – even death – can occur, especially in anyone living in a hot or dry climate.

Living with LND and KSS

These tests for LND and KSS are all very well, but there doesn't seem to be any prospect of curing the children with these metabolic disorders, does there? What have we gained now that we know our two sons have KSS, for example?

You now have an end to the time-consuming tests, inconvenience and uncertainty before the correct diagnosis was given – this is important to families and to health services. Now you can concentrate on getting a realistic assessment of future possibilities for the boys. In addition, you can ask for an accurate test to identify the faulty gene that underlies your sons' condition; this test, and genetic counselling, will also help other carriers in your family who are hoping to have children.

Although there is currently no cure for the nervous system disorders in LND and its variants, the important point for parents is that KSS has no associated cerebral palsy and is treatable with allopurinol. However, as in LND, allopurinol must be given with care and your boys should be monitored to determine the correct dose and to prevent a build-up of xanthine instead in their kidneys.

After having had a son with LND, my wife was pregnant again and we were told that we could have a prenatal test of a chorionic villus sample (CVS) at 12 weeks. What is this test, and how does it work?

This test involves taking a tiny sample of tissue from the placenta, by a careful biopsy using a special 'imaging' technique to follow the placing of the instrument. The tissue sample is then carefully examined and tested to see if the enzyme activity (HPRT activity) is normal, low or absent, and for the sex of the developing baby. A low level or absence of the HPRT activity would be cause for concern, and, if the sex is male, you may decide to think about terminating the pregnancy.

We had the CVS test 12 weeks into the pregnancy and were told that, although the unborn baby was male, HPRT enzyme activity was normal. We agreed, with some misgiving, to proceed to a further check at 18 weeks, when normal enzyme was confirmed. Our healthy baby boy was born and normal enzyme confirmed again, but we were shattered when we suddenly started to find the same orange crystals as we had found on his brother's nappies. What has gone wrong?

Nothing is wrong. All newborn babies produce and excrete a lot of uric acid in the first week or two of life; this is because the ability of their kidneys to reabsorb uric acid is not yet functioning properly. It is the *persistent* presence of these crystals in the nappies over the next month or months that should ring alarm bells for parents (when 'failure to thrive' will also become evident). This is unlikely to have happened with your new son, because the HPRT activity tested normal at three different times. (Note: in a similar instance we know of, the healthy younger boy is now 10 years old and helps his older brother with such activities as Riding for the Disabled and setting up his special bicycle.)

My son, who has LND, cannot walk or talk and needs a lot of care. Can we get help with nursing on a regular basis?

See your GP to find out what help is available in your area. If your son is chronically ill and requires the help of another person in connection with 'bodily functions' – feeding, washing, toileting – or taking medicines, over and above the help that would be expected to be required by a normal child of the same age, he is probably eligible to receive the Care Component of the Disability Living Allowance (DLA). This is available to children of any age. If he has problems with getting about outdoors (such that he is unable or virtually unable to walk), he should be eligible to receive the Mobility Component of DLA, provided he is 3 years of age or more at the time the application is made. DLA is meant to help with the extra costs of being disabled. The money can be used to purchase extra nursing care if that is what you want, or for any other purpose for that matter. Home nursing care is, of course, also available on the NHS and is accessed via your GP.

Our son's illness means he needs (and gets) a lot of attention, but I feel that his older sister is thus being deprived of attention. What can we do if we want to take his sister on an outing or have a holiday?

Ask your GP or health visitor to help you find some respite care. Facilities for caring for your son for periods ranging from a few hours to a week or two will vary according to where you live, as local councils usually depend heavily on voluntary organisations. Some organisations for the disabled offer carers who come to your home – the local council may be able to help here – and some children's hospices offer respite care for children with severe disorders of the nervous system. A list is available from the Association of Children's Hospices (contact details in Appendix 1, ***Useful addresses***).

Our son is now taking allopurinol. Will it help with the other aspects of these metabolic disorders?

Children with LND, KSS or PRPS respond very rapidly to allopurinol, but the drug treats only the accumulation of urate and so has no effect on the 'non-gout' symptoms. Provided that the allopurinol dose is not too high, it will help protect the kidneys from damage or from further damage. With allopurinol the high levels of uric acid are replaced by a related chemical, xanthine, which is much less soluble than uric acid, so it is essential to keep the dose as low as practicable. It is essential, too, that he takes lots of fluid, to prevent deposits of uric acid from forming. Uric acid is less soluble when the urine is acid, but solubility can be increased 12-fold by taking alkalinising tablets (or liquid potassium citrate disguised with orange juice; see Chapter 3, ***Drugs to combat the pain and inflammation***) together with the allopurinol.

It may be useful to consult the diet advice in Chapter 5 (***Food and drink***), and to avoid foods high in purines, but remember not to restrict protein or calories in growing children.

I was asked not to allow my son to have chocolate biscuits or puddings and drinks such as cola or Lucozade for three days before he gives a sample to the laboratory. Should I always restrict his intake of these things?

No, this was just to help the laboratory make a clear diagnosis from the urine test. Caffeine and related molecules are present in all the foods you mentioned, and these chemicals resemble the molecules that are analysed in blood and urine samples. Because the genetic changes in disorders such as LND and PRPS have sometimes led to small but characteristic alterations in the concentration of these important chemicals (nucleotides and uric acid), it is essential to have a sample that is free from caffeine and similar molecules that could give confusing results.

In addition to the foods you mentioned, don't let your son drink tea or coffee before the blood test. Please don't give your son any 'cold cures' that contain caffeine (it is not normally present in children's formulations) and don't let well-meaning friends give him chocolate to comfort him before taking the sample.

See Table 5.1 for a list of purine-rich foods to be avoided routinely in all the metabolic disorders described in this chapter.

My toddler has not really grown as we would expect and he has been having some fits recently. My doctor thought we should get a blood sample tested for one of these metabolic disorders, and the result came back that the level of uric acid in the sample was lower than expected. What does this mean? What other tests can be done to find out what the problem is?

Usually you would be asked to supply urine as well as blood for these initial diagnostic tests. A low plasma urate level in your son could be caused by a low-purine diet or by a defect in the xanthine oxidase enzyme. Alternatively, some factor may be encouraging the excretion of uric acid into the urine. Assuming your child has not been taking any prescribed drugs, we would be interested to know if you have been giving him any dietary supplements, for example high-dose vitamin C tablets, which will speed up the excretion of uric acid and would give a low plasma urate value in most people.

If the urine is tested as well, it may show that he is producing too much uric acid, which is being excreted. So a low level in plasma and a high level in urine would tell us that, although the body is making a good deal of uric acid, it is being excreted very efficiently. Your doctor should ask for uric acid to be measured in both blood and urine, and for enzymes to be measured in red blood cells by a specialist unit. A defective enzyme could explain a high production of urate, but whether the urate is higher in the plasma or the urine depends on the relative rate of excretion – which is more efficient in all children (as described earlier in this chapter). It is important to stop any vitamin supplement a few days before beginning the collection of these samples.

7

Research and the future

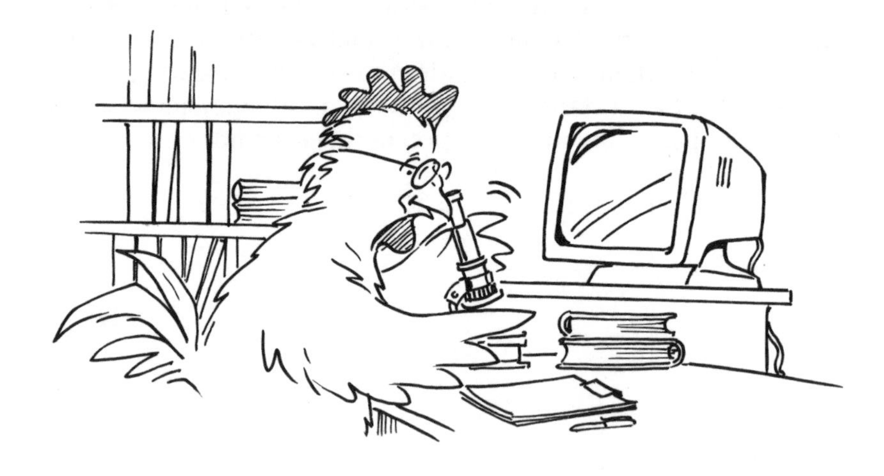

People with gout are no longer condemned to live with a recurring painful condition and ultimately with permanent disability. Biochemists have investigated the metabolic pathways through which uric acid passes as it is manufactured in the body, and several effective drugs now allow us to control the production of uric acid (allopurinol) and its excretion from the kidneys (probenecid, sulfinpyrazone, benzbromarone) so most people with gout can now lead a reasonably normal life. Remember that part of the remedy is up to you – equally vital factors in controlling uric acid levels are weight loss or maintenance of an already healthy weight, avoidance of purine-rich foods and beverages, and rigorous control of your blood pressure.

For people with the inherited disorders described in Chapter 6 (***Gout in young people***), the important first step is accurate diagnosis. Modern molecular genetic techniques can identify the tiny changes in our genes that may lead to both small and large changes in the concentrations of the essential chemicals in our blood. With this knowledge, parents can discuss the likelihood of having another affected child, and the options for treatment of existing affected children.

Can gout be cured?

After all these centuries, why can't gout be properly cured?

Classic primary gout in men is the result of an inherited defect or difference that appears at puberty, and means that their kidneys reabsorb less uric acid from their urine than do women's. It is a fact of life! In adult men, urate already circulates at levels close to the maximum before crystals will form. When levels of urate in the blood reach saturation point (around 420 micromoles per litre, 7mg/100ml) excess uric acid from the diet will then just tip the scales towards gouty arthritis. In other words, it is part of the human condition, and perhaps will never be 'cured' in the way that infectious diseases are eliminated.

We can certainly look for good management of the symptoms using drugs and modern advice on 'healthy eating', without repeating the stringent food rationing that caused the disappearance of this type of gout during the two world wars in the 20th century. The possibility of gene manipulation is sometimes mentioned as a possible answer to some disorders but, in the case of classic gout, such efforts can be difficult to justify when most cases are managed well through a combination of a low-purine diet, regular allopurinol and the control of weight and blood pressure.

Are any new drugs being developed for gout?

Allopurinol has been very successful since its introduction for gout. It is the cheapest and most effective drug used specifically to treat hyperuricaemia. Allopurinol inhibits the xanthine oxidase enzyme, but it is slowly converted to a similar molecule, oxypurinol, which can cause some serious reactions in a very small number of susceptible people with inefficient kidneys. Some newly developed chemicals (without this side-effect) have been studied in the laboratory but it may be some time before they supersede the general benefit of allopurinol.

When some cancers of the white blood cells, such as non-Hodgkin's lymphoma or acute lymphocytic leukaemia, are treated with drugs that kill the rapidly dividing cells, the blood system acquires a huge burden of natural compounds released from the cancer cells. This is known as the 'tumour lysis syndrome', characterised by hyperuricaemia, leading to complications including renal failure. People undergoing chemotherapy for these cancers are routinely treated with allopurinol before the therapy begins, and with fluids to encourage the excretion of uric acid from the kidneys. Recently a new treatment has been investigated, using preparations of the enzyme uricase, or urate oxidase, which is found in most other species of mammals, and which converts uric acid into a molecule that can be excreted more easily. Injections of the enzyme into the muscles or the veins lead to a rapid decline of the plasma urate levels – within hours rather than days. The enzyme treatment is used for five to seven days, allowing cancer drugs to be started within that time with no danger of renal failure. It should be stressed that this treatment is very expensive, and not without its own potential side-effects, so it cannot be used as a routine way to keep hyperuricaemia at bay. It is currently offered only at specialist cancer centres for people with a vigorous cancer.

For people with classic gout, perhaps complicated by high blood pressure or being overweight, a recent addition to the drugs used to treat high blood pressure, losartan (which acts by inhibiting the enzyme angiotensin-II), also increases elimination of uric acid by the kidneys. Combined with allopurinol, it has been very effective in lowering plasma uric acid even further, as well as controlling hypertension, in people with FJHN. A drug called fenofibrate, prescribed to decrease the levels of cholesterol in the blood, has a similar action.

Research into metabolic gout

What research is being directed at the purine metabolic disorders?

Not enough, we believe. Unfortunately, these disorders are considered too rare and cannot compete for research funds in the current climate, which favours large projects addressing diseases that affect many people, such as cancer or heart disease. Many scientists involved in their diagnosis struggle to keep research alive. Research is typically carried out in medical schools and hospitals, where patients can be studied but where resources may be stretched, rather than in laboratories funded by pharmaceutical companies.

It may be a small comfort to know that people who have rare genetic disorders such as those described in Chapter 6 are nature's valuable mistakes, telling us what can happen when the normal system 'goes wrong'. Cells from patients may be used in the laboratory for scientists to identify the defective steps in the metabolic pathways. Synthetic compounds may be devised either to inhibit a step or to enhance its activity, in a process of the design or discovery of new drugs. Some pharmaceutical companies use collections of potentially useful chemicals, testing them against cells in culture, and in these studies the cells from people with different disorders could be invaluable.

Have the guilty genes for gout been identified?

Not yet. Certainly in FJHN several genes are involved. One mutation has been found in three large families world-wide, another in only one. At least 11 other FJHN families do not have either mutation. The other defective genes remain elusive but finding them could lead to the guilty genes for classic gout being revealed as well. Now that scientific methods can give us information on the genes and enzymes involved in metabolic pathways, all that is needed is money and improved technology, which may become more available as classic gout becomes one of the diseases of plenty in the West.

I am a doctor in China, where primary gout is still uncommon. I recently met a young boy and his sister, both of whom have painful, distorted knee joints (Figure 7.1). We took some fluid from the joints and found a very large amount of crystals; plasma urate levels were also very high. The children are of normal intelligence, they do not have cerebral palsy, nor do they have any problems with their movements. Is this is a metabolic disorder like those you described in Chapter 6?

This is a recent example of the intriguing enquiries that occasionally reach a specialist centre. It is interesting that a girl is

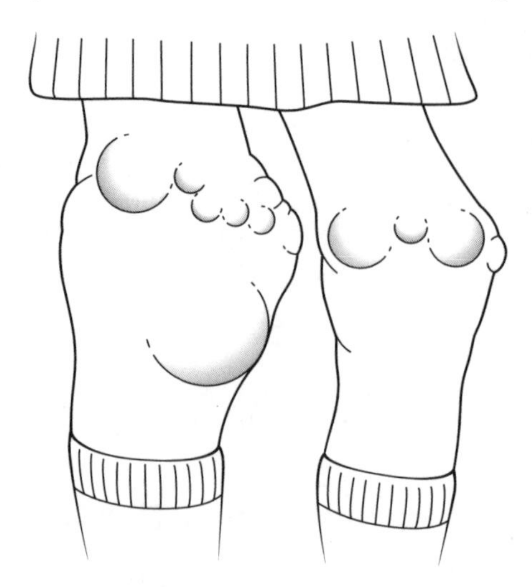

Figure 7.1 Swollen and disfigured knee joints in a young girl with an undiagnosed disorder that includes gout and hyperuricaemia.

affected, as this is not common with the 'X-linked' disorders. However, female carriers in PRPS do develop gout, so this could be the first family showing very early onset in the female as well. Someone with FJHN might have been expected to have some kidney damage before gout symptoms were apparent. In this example, the specialist unit would ask for samples of blood and urine to measure the suspect enzymes as well as the amount of uric acid and the various purines that are found in body fluids. It is always possible that these children may be the first reported cases of a previously unknown disorder, picked up by an astute doctor with a special interest in gout – as has been the case for many genetic disorders, including LND.

Help for people with gout

Now that we are on-line at home, I have been looking up gout on the internet. There seem to be many websites with information on health, but often I find that they give advice that conflicts with the next site I visit. How do I know which is correct?

It is so much easier to search for information in this way rather than rummaging through books in a library or bookshop, and we can find ourselves snowed under with information. Not all of it is trustworthy, and some may be only personal opinions of one writer – but this is the case with some magazine articles too. Be aware that scientific publications are also superseded as new information emerges, and thus scientific papers quoted in corroboration may be out of date by now. You will be well advised to take the information on many websites with a pinch of salt, especially where commercial advertising is concerned, and you will also find that reputable websites (e.g. those listed in the website section of Appendix 1, ***Useful addresses***) are reliable and accurate. You might find *The Patient's Internet Handbook* useful when searching for reliable information (details in Appendix 2, ***Useful publications***).

I want to leave a legacy to an appropriate charity that will specifically help people with gout. Can you recommend one?

Supporting the research into the purine metabolic disorders would be immensely helpful for sufferers and researchers alike. Please ask PUMPA (contact details in Appendix 1, ***Useful addresses***) for information about this.

Can I offer my services to a voluntary group that supports children with metabolic disorders?

Your local council or health authority may be able to put you in touch with a group that organises Saturday clubs for disabled teenagers or respite care for families. The Department of Medicine or of Paediatrics in some hospitals may know of facilities used by some of their patients. The only groups that specifically handle LND patients are PUMPA and CLIMB; the organisation Contact a Family may be able to give you more general ideas (contact details in Appendix 1, ***Useful addresses***). You may also find information about organisations in your area listed in your local library.

I live in Germany at present. Where can I get help or diagnosis for a suspected disorder?

Advice and, where possible, help from PUMPA is available to all of Europe on their website (see Appendix 1, ***Useful addresses***), set up through a project sponsored by the European Community (BMH4-CT98-3079). When the project began, comprehensive diagnostic facilities were available in only four countries; they are now provided in 19 countries.

A directory of the laboratories offering these diagnostic facilities throughout Europe, as a result of an EC-funded collaboration, is also available on the website for the European Society for the Study of Purine and Pyrimidine Metabolism in Man (ESSPPMM; see Appendix 1 for the website).

Help from other families can be very valuable when a child is newly diagnosed with a metabolic disorder. The PUMPA website includes links to a European federation for Lesch–Nyhan patients, linking families in Spain, France and Italy, and other groups will be added as they make themselves known. Some other addresses are given in Appendix 1.

Glossary

Words in *italic* in the definitions are also defined in this Glossary.

acupuncture A traditional Chinese system of relieving pain by inserting fine needles beneath the skin. The needles are thought to stimulate sensory nerves, which cause the release of the body's natural pain-killers into the circulation. Therefore the needles may be inserted at a different site from the source of the pain.

acute A word meaning 'sharp' – thus it describes a condition where the symptoms appear rapidly and are severe or painful. In *gout*, the acute attack has a brief duration compared with *chronic* (long-term) accumulation of *uric acid*.

adenine/adenosine Adenine is one of the nitrogen-containing bases, or *purines*, that occur in the *nucleic acids* DNA and RNA in all cells. Adenosine is a related chemical. (See also *ATP*.)

addiction Physical dependence on a drug that is taken regularly – leading to unpleasant 'withdrawal symptoms' when the drug is stopped. This term is also often used when the dependence is psychological. In each case the drug should be withdrawn gradually.

allergic reaction An over-reaction of the body's immune system to a foreign particle or chemical. When the body encounters the trigger again, its reactions can range from mild symptoms resembling hay-fever to severe inflammation, dermatitis and shock.

allopurinol A drug that acts to reduce the levels of *uric acid* formed from *purines* in the body. The tablets may be generic allopurinol, or provided under the trade names Hamarin or Zyloric.

ampicillin An *antibiotic*, one of the penicillin group.

analgesic A pain-killing drug, such as aspirin, paracetamol, *NSAIDs*, narcotics. (See also *COX-2 inhibitors*.)

antibiotic A drug that can kill bacteria without harming the patient (unless he or she is allergic to it); for example, penicillins, tetracyclines, aminoglycosides, cephalosporins.

anti-inflammatory drugs Drugs that react against the various causes of inflammation. For *gout*, the *corticosteroid* drugs and *colchicine* are useful anti-inflammatories. *NSAIDs* also act as pain-killers where the inflammation is the cause of the pain, by inhibiting the *cyclo-oxygenase enzymes* (COX-1 and *COX-2*).

arthritis Inflammation of one or more joints, resulting in pain, heat, swelling and redness over the affected joint, whose movement will be restricted. There are many types of arthritis, including rheumatoid arthritis, ankylosing spondylitis, infectious (or septic) or reactive arthritis, degenerative ('wear and tear') conditions such as *osteoarthritis*, and *metabolic* forms of arthritis such as *gout*.

ATP Adenosine triphosphate, a *purine*-containing compound that is needed in all cells to store chemical energy, for the conversion of small molecules into other material, and for the contraction of muscle. About half the *uric acid* excreted through the kidneys is derived from ATP.

back-pressure This refers to a build-up of pressure in the kidneys that occurs when the outflow of urine is obstructed, for example when the prostate is enlarged or when stones are found in the *ureter* or in the bladder itself. This increased pressure in the kidney, called hydronephrosis, may result in kidney failure.

benzbromarone (Desuric) A *uricosuric drug*; it is ten times more potent than probenecid, which was for many years the most widely used uricosuric drug. Unlike probenecid, it can be prescribed for people with kidney damage.

bronchodilator A drug that can cause the muscles around the air passages to relax, thus relieving the symptoms of asthma.

caffeine A stimulant and mild *diuretic* that is found in coffee, tea and some over-the-counter preparations sold as pain-killers and for the relief of cold symptoms. Some canned soft drinks contain caffeine: e.g. Coca-Cola, PepsiCola, Lucozade, Red Bull. If it is present, caffeine will always be noted on the label of packaged drinks and pain-killers.

calorie-controlled diet An effective way to lose weight, provided it is accompanied by will-power and increased physical activity. The simplest way to cut calories is to eat smaller portions of your regular diet but, because fatty foods contribute calories in the most concentrated form, cutting fats will be most effective. Low-carbohydrate diets are now being recommended more frequently, because they help to control the symptoms of Type 2 *diabetes*.

cerebral palsy A disorder, with a variety of causes, appearing before the age of three years and affecting the voluntary movements (walking, talking, manipulation). *Lesch–Nyhan disease* (LND) is an inherited form of cerebral palsy caused by the defect in *HPRT* activity.

chemotherapy The use of chemicals to cure or to manage a disease. Usually the term refers to treatment of cancer with drugs that kill cancer cells, contrasting with radiotherapy (using x-rays).

chondrocalcinosis The presence of crystals of calcium pyrophosphate dihydrate within the cartilage in the joint (typically the knee). Also known as pyrophosphate arthropathy or pseudo-gout when inflammation occurs.

choreo-athetosis A disorder of movement in which the person weaves irregularly and sways like a dancer. The movements are involuntary. (See also *cerebral palsy.*)

chronic A term that describes a condition with a gradual onset and slow changes over a long time. Such a condition may or may not be severe or life-threatening. In *gout*, the chronic condition may also have *acute* episodes that have broadly the same cause.

chronic tophaceous gout Long-standing *gout* in which tophi (singular *tophus*) are deposited in and around joints. In some people, the tophi are the principal symptom, and there is little *arthritis* pain.

colchicine A drug derived from the autumn crocus plant, colchicum. It is effective in relieving the pain of gouty *arthritis* attacks.

corticosteroid Naturally occurring chemicals (hormones) produced by the adrenal glands, or synthetic drugs with similar chemical structures and effects. The drugs are powerful *anti-inflammatory* agents. (Also called 'steroids', which should not be confused with anabolic steroids sometimes used illegally by athletes to build up their muscular strength.)

COX-2 inhibitors Drugs that inhibit the action of the enzyme *cyclo-oxygenase*-2 and thus relieve pain caused by inflammation. Their advantage over other (COX-1) *NSAIDs* is the reduced effect on the stomach, lowering the risk of gastric ulcers or bleeding in the stomach. Despite the higher cost of COX-2 inhibitors, the National Institute for Clinical Excellence (NICE) recommends their use for extreme and chronic pain caused by inflammation, where the patient is susceptible to the gastric effects of NSAIDs.

CVS Chorionic villus sampling. After the ninth week of pregnancy, a tiny sample of cells is removed from the part of the placenta provided by the fetus. The cells are studied to determine if there are any abnormalities in the chromosomes or *enzymes*, which would imply a disorder in the developing baby.

cyclo-oxygenase An *enzyme* that is part of the body's inflammatory response. Inhibiting either form of this enzyme (COX-1 or *COX-2*) therefore helps to relieve the pain of inflammation.

degenerative diseases Conditions that occur in later life, partly caused by wear and tear in the body, such as *osteoarthritis*, Type 2 *diabetes* and *hypertension* (high blood pressure).

diabetes This term usually refers to diabetes mellitus, of which there are two main types. Type 1 diabetes occurs in childhood or adolescence in people who cannot make enough of the hormone insulin to control the body's use of sugars and carbohydrate food. The condition is severe but it can be controlled by injections of insulin. Type 2 diabetes typically occurs after the age of 40 in people whose body responds inadequately to insulin. Drugs or insulin may be given, but emphasis is also placed on a healthy diet, with weight reduction if appropriate.

diuretics Drugs that promote the excretion of salts and water from the kidney, and therefore often referred to as 'water tablets'. They are usually prescribed to reduce oedema (puffiness) around the ankles and lower legs that may be caused by any of several disorders. When levels of *uric acid* in the kidney are high, some diuretics (e.g. thiazides such as bendrofluazide) are known to interfere with its excretion into the urine, resulting in high levels in the blood.

DNA Deoxyribonucleic acid, a very large molecule in the nucleus of all cells. DNA is especially important in cells that are dividing, because it contains the information (genetic code) that will enable cells to carry out their functions, in particular to divide and produce another cell of identical *genetic* composition, and to manufacture *enzymes* and structural components of the cells.

drug interaction Two or more drugs taken together can cause a loss in potency, an increase in potency, or alter the period during which one of the drugs is active. Some drug interactions alter the speed or efficiency of natural processes, such as the excretion of *uric acid* from the kidneys.

enzymes Protein molecules in all cells of our body, and in our digestive system and the blood circulation, that carry out chemical reactions. Because each enzyme has a very specific structure, related to the reaction it carries out, drugs can be designed to knock out the action of one enzyme. This is the basis of *allopurinol*'s effect on the production of *uric acid.*

FJGN or **FJHN** Familial juvenile gouty/hyperuricaemic *nephropathy*. A condition affecting children and young men and women, characterised by kidney failure if it is not recognised and treated. The kidney symptoms are always accompanied by high levels of *uric acid* in the blood, which often results in *tophaceous gout.*

gastric ulcer An open sore in the lining of the stomach, which may fail to heal unless treated. The acid juices in the stomach, digestive *enzyme*s and bile, act on the mucous lining of the stomach to form ulcers, but taking *NSAID*s or *corticosteroids* can increase the risk.

gastritis Inflammation of the lining of the stomach, which may precede ulcers.

genetic/genetic code Referring to the inheritance of characteristics from parents. The genetic code is a chemical means of transferring information from the DNA of the chromosomes. This information can be transmitted to the cells that will become eggs and sperm, or can be used in each cell of the body to make the proteins that will contribute to the eventual shape and function of the body.

genetic counselling Advice given to parents who wish to consider the likelihood that an inherited disorder will affect their children.

Usually parents will know that one carries the faulty gene, or they may already have one child with such a disorder and will need to think about the options for diagnosing an affected child before birth (see *prenatal diagnosis*), or for terminating the pregnancy.

gout A disease resulting from the accumulation of *uric acid* in the blood and the formation of crystals of *sodium urate* in the joints. The acute phase – gouty arthritis – is a painful attack of *arthritis*, usually in the big toe, with a very rapid onset. *Chronic* gout may include the deposition of urate salts as *tophi* in the skin, bone and cartilage, and high levels of uric acid may damage the kidneys. With modern drug treatment and diet, primary gout can be well controlled. Rare defects in the *metabolism* of *purines*, or a familial *nephropathy*, may also be associated with gout symptoms. (See also *primary gout* and *secondary gout*.)

GP General practitioner; family doctor.

guanine/guanosine Guanine is one of the nitrogen-containing bases, or *purines*, that occurs in the *nucleic acids* DNA and RNA in all cells. Guanosine is a related chemical, found in beer.

HPRT Abbreviation for the *enzyme* hypoxanthine-guanine phosphoribosyltransferase, which carries out a crucial reaction in the recycling of *purines* from daily wear and tear in the body. Complete lack of HPRT will result in *Lesch–Nyhan disease* (LND), while partial deficiency of the activity will lead to the symptoms of *LND variant* or *KSS*. The gene for HPRT is carried on the *X chromosome*, so these conditions are usually seen only in boys.

HRT Hormone replacement therapy: usually refers to female steroid hormones given to women who have passed the menopause.

hypertension High blood pressure. There are many causes, including narrowing of the renal artery, and many complications, including renal failure. Combinations of drugs (anti-hypertensives) may be used to control the blood pressure, and weight loss may also be advised.

hyperuricaemia An abnormally high level of *uric acid* or urate salts in the blood. This may be caused by reabsorption of uric acid in inefficient kidneys, or may result from high levels of uric acid as *purines* are *metabolised* for excretion.

hyperuricosuria/hyperuricuria An abnormally high level of *uric acid* in the urine. It may be caused by efficient excretion of uric acid, made from a high concentration of *purines* in the diet or from our cells. The concentration of uric acid in the blood should also be measured for comparison.

Kelley–Seegmiller syndrome (KSS) A *metabolic* disorder resulting in over-production of *purines*, for the same reason as *Lesch–Nyhan disease* (LND). In KSS, the *enzyme HPRT* is defective rather than completely absent, so affected boys do not have any of the problems in the central nervous system as found in LND. The first indication that a boy has KSS may be *acute* renal failure after an infection, dehydration or the use of antibiotics, all of which increase the concentration of *uric acid* in the kidneys. The principal long-term concerns are gouty *arthritis* and *kidney stones*, both of which can be prevented by treatmentwith *allopurinol.*

kidney stones (renal calculi) Hard masses formed in the kidney tubules from insoluble material that becomes concentrated during the excretion processes taking place in the kidneys. The most commonly found kidney stones are composed of calcium oxalate. *Uric acid* stones may be formed when *hyperuricosuria* has been present for several years. Stones may cause pain, but often there are no symptoms until the kidney tubules become blocked. If the flow of urine is obstructed, there is a danger of infection in the urinary tract and the kidney(s).

Lesch–Nyhan disease/syndrome (LND/LNS) A *metabolic* disorder resulting in over-production of *purines*, and thus in high levels of *uric acid.* The gene coding for the *enzyme* is inherited on the *X chromosome*, and, because boys have only one X chromosome, the condition affects boys who lack the only copy of the gene on their single X chromosome. Their mother and sisters may lack one copy or carry one defective copy of the gene with no apparent ill-effect. Affected children have *gout*, increased muscular activity, with poor co-ordination and involuntary, jerky movements, and a distressing compulsion to bite or scratch themselves (self-mutilation). The gout can be controlled with *allopurinol.*

LND variants Boys with an LND variant have milder symptoms in the nervous system than with *Lesch–Nyhan disease* but the same over-production of *uric acid.*

lithaemia Another term for *hyperuricaemia.*

lithiasis Stones (which may be composed of various insoluble compounds – e.g. oxalic acid, xanthine and *uric acid*, singly or together) deposited in the kidneys, urinary tract, gall-bladder, etc.

metabolic/metabolism Concerning the reactions in the body that convert food and other chemicals to provide energy and raw materials in the body's cells. Also includes the reactions that re-use or excrete substances.

monoarticular Occurring in only one joint (e.g. gouty *arthritis* may occur in the big toe of one foot).

nephrologist A specialist in the study and management of kidney disorders.

nephropathy Disorder of the kidneys, often involving impaired excretion and/or kidney stones.

NSAID. Non-steroidal anti-inflammatory drug. See Table 3.1.

nucleic acids (DNA and RNA) Very large molecules whose structure contains and transmits *genetic* information.

obesity Accumulation of fat in the body, giving a final body weight that is at least 20 per cent higher than recommended for the person's height and build.

osteoarthritis Degenerative damage caused by wear on the cartilage in joints, especially load-bearing or damaged joints. The pain and stiffness progress slowly and chronically, and movement may be restricted.

pH A measure of the acidity (low pH values) or the alkalinity (high pH values) of a solution. Pure water has a neutral pH value of 7.0.

plasma (blood plasma) The yellowish liquid part of blood. The plasma can be separated from the blood cells, and the presence of components such as antibodies, salts and trace elements can be measured. When measuring the concentration of *sodium urate* in the blood, the resulting figure is the 'plasma urate level'.

podagra Gouty *arthritis* in the joints of the foot.

podiatrist Specialist in the care of feet; formerly or also known as a chiropodist. Podiatrists may perform minor foot surgery and may prescribe treatment for gouty *arthritis.*

polarised light, polarising microscope When light waves pass through a transparent medium that causes them to vibrate in only one plane, the light is described as 'polarised'. This is the same as the anti-glare effect found with polarised sunglasses. Just as car windscreens and waterfalls can look different when wearing these sunglasses, crystals can show brilliant rainbow-like effects when seen under polarised light in the microscope. The distinctive appearance of crystals of *sodium urate* under polarised light can be used to differentiate them from other crystal deposits, such as calcium pyrophosphate dihydrate, that might be found in joints or in the kidneys.

polyarticular (*Arthritis*) occurring in several joints.

prenatal diagnosis Testing to check for the possible presence of a *genetic* problem in the fetus. The methods used are chorionic villus sampling (*CVS*) in the first three months, or amniocentesis/chordocentesis in the third to sixth months. These tests take tiny samples of cells or blood from the developing fetus.

primary gout *Gout* caused by high levels of *uric acid* in the blood of middle-aged men, which arise either from the diet or from a natural over-production of *purines*.

protein Essential components of all living organisms, as *enzymes*, as hormones or as structural components. Proteins are composed of the smaller amino acids, which are in turn obtained by recycling proteins in the diet.

pseudo-gout see *chondrocalcinosis*

puberty The transition between childhood and adulthood, accompanied by numerous physical changes and the development of the internal and external sex organs.

purine Natural chemical containing nitrogen, carbon, hydrogen and oxygen forming a 'base' (*adenine* or *guanine*). When attached to a sugar and phosphate groups, a *purine nucleotide* is formed. Purine molecules are released by breakdown of *nucleic acids*, and are converted into *uric acid* by the *enzymes* in the liver.

purine nucleotides The single molecules of adenosine and guanosine phosphates (see *ATP*); they take part in the *metabolic* reactions in the cells, and are also used in constructing the *nucleic acids*.

renal calculi see *kidney stones*

renal failure Failure of the kidneys to continue filtering or excreting urine; it may be *acute* or *chronic.*

rheumatologist A specialist in the study and management of disorders of joints, bones, muscles and ligaments.

RNA see *nucleic acids*

secondary gout *Gout* caused by another disease or induced by a drug. (See Chapter 1.)

sodium urate The salt of *uric acid*, which accumulates in tophi (singular *tophus*) or as crystalline deposits in the joints.

solubility The extent to which a salt or other chemical compound can be dissolved in water or body fluids. As more of a chemical is added to the fluid, it becomes a 'saturated solution', in which no more can dissolve; crystals or other deposits may then begin to form. Solubility may be affected by the acidity of the solution; for example, *uric acid* is less soluble when the urine is more acid than usual.

steroid see *corticosteroid*

synovial fluid Fluid in the space between the two parts of a moving joint (i.e. within the cavity of a joint).

theophylline A compound from the leaves of the tea plant, it relaxes smooth muscles such as those in the breathing passages or blood vessels. It can be used to control bronchial asthma.

tophaceous gout The presence of tophi (singular *tophus*) may be the only evidence of *gout* in some people, such as older women taking *diuretic* therapy or boys with *Lesch–Nyhan disease.* (See also *chronic tophaceous gout.*)

tophus (plural = tophi) A solid deposit of *sodium urate* and membranous structures, typically under the skin or in the ear cartilage. They may reflect sites of earlier damage to joints of the fingers or toes or other parts of the skeleton such as the elbows or knees. Rarely, a deposit may be found in the vertebrae.

ureter The tube connecting the kidney to the bladder, and hence transporting urine to the bladder.

urolithiasis Stones (derived mainly from insoluble deposits of *uric acid*) in the urinary tract.

uric acid The end-product of the reactions that break down *purines* in humans. Uric acid is excreted through the kidneys and also through the gut, in bile. The salts of uric acid (urate compounds) are insoluble, hence their tendency to form crystals.

uricase/urate oxidase This *enzyme* is found naturally in all mammals except for man, the higher apes and some breeds of dog. It converts *uric acid* to a more soluble compound, allantoin, with the release of a molecule of hydrogen peroxide. Human physiology has adapted well to the lack of the enzyme; uricase may only be really necessary when there is an urgent need to reduce the concentration of urate in the blood of cancer patients.

uricosuric drugs Drugs that help to promote the excretion of *uric acid* in the urine by preventing the reabsorption of uric acid into the blood in the kidneys.

vegetarian diet A diet that excludes animal meat and usually also fish. Most vegetarian diets allow dairy products because animals have not been killed, but vegans eat no food that is connected with animals. A vegan diet is often deficient in vitamin B_{12}.

X chromosome One of the 'sex' chromosomes. Women have a pair of X chromosomes, while men have one X and one Y. The genes for some sex-specific stages in development are found on the Y chromosome, so they determine whether the child will be a boy or a girl.

X-linked disorder When one of the genes on the *X chromosome* is faulty, a boy who carries it will be affected, because he has only the faulty copy and thus a defective *enzyme* is made. A girl will usually be helped by the presence of an intact copy of the gene on her other X chromosome, allowing 'good' enzyme to be made. Diagrams are given in Chapter 6 (***Gout in young people***).

xanthine An intermediate in the breakdown of *adenosine* and *guanine* to *uric acid*. Xanthine concentrations will rise when *allopurinol* blocks the *enzyme* reaction that should produce uric acid.

xanthine oxidase The *enzyme* that usually breaks down *xanthine* to form *uric acid*. This enzyme is inhibited by *allopurinol* to varying degrees depending on the dose.

Appendix 1
Useful Addresses

For patients and their families

Arthritis Care
18 Stephenson Way
London NW1 2HD
Tel: 020 7916 1500
Fax: 020 7380 6505
Helpline: 0808 800 4050
(Monday–Friday 12–4p.m.)
Website:
www.arthritiscare.org.uk
Provides information, counselling, training and social contact. The first port of call for anyone with arthritis, including gout. There are many smaller organisations for particular types of arthritis; the helpline can provide details.

Arthritis Research Campaign
Copeman House
St Mary's Court
St Mary's Gate
Chesterfield S41 7TD
Tel: 01246 558033
Fax: 01246 558007
Website: www.arc.org.uk
The leading arthritis research organisation in the UK, funding much research and producing useful information (including a booklet on gout) for patients.

Association of Children's Hospices
Kings House
14 Orchard Street
Bristol BS1 5EH
Tel: 0117 905 5082
Fax: 0117 905 5340
Website:
www.childhospice.org.uk
An 'umbrella' support group, providing information on hospices especially for children, respite care and home services; links to other organisations for children.

Chailey Heritage Clinical Services
Beggars Wood Road
North Chailey
East Sussex BN8 4JN
Tel: 0182 572 2112
Fax: 0182 572 4700
Website:
www.southdowns.nhs.uk/caring
Specialised rehabilitation services for children with severe disability, including LND.

Children in Scotland
5 Shandwick Place
Edinburgh EH2 4RG
Tel: 0131 228 8484
Fax: 0131 228 8585
Website:
www.childreninscotland.org.uk
An independent charity and national agency for over 300 organisations working on behalf of Scottish children and families.

Children's Trust
Tadworth Court
Tadworth
Surrey KT20 5RU
Tel: 01737 365000
Fax: 01737 365012
Website:
www.the childrenstrust.org.uk
Offers long- and short-term respite care and nursing help for profoundly disabled children and children with brain injuries.

CLIMB – Children living with inherited metabolic diseases
The Quadrangle
Crewe Hall
Weston Road
Crewe CW1 6UR
Tel: 0870 7700 326
Website: www.climb.org.uk
Offers information and support to families, carers and professionals, and links to other groups. Also funds research into metabolic diseases.

Contact a Family
209–212 City Road
London EC1V 1JN
Tel: 020 7608 8700
Fax: 020 7608 8701
Helpline: 0808 808 3555
Website: www.cafamily.org.uk
Offers information on over 1,000 rare disorders and links to other groups. Can put families in touch with each other and with counselling services. A Directory, updated annually, is also available at £35 in hard copy.

Crossroads Caring for Carers
10 Regent Place
Rugby
Warwickshire CV21 2PN
Tel: England: 01788 573653
Wales: 02920 222282
Scotland: 0141 226 3793
Fax: (England): 01788 565498
Website: www.crossroads.org.uk
Co-ordinates local schemes for home-based support for carers, and trained care assistants to provide respite. Supports and delivers high-quality services for carers and people with care needs via its local branches.

INS (Integrated Neurological Services)
42 Alexandra Road
Kew, Richmond
Surrey TW9 2BS
Tel/Fax: 020 8940 7662
Email: ekinnear@ins.org.uk
Physiotherapists-led self-help groups helping people with neurological conditions to meet and exchange coping strategies.

Lesch–Nyhan Registry
Email: LNSIA@yahoogroups.com
Website:
www.64.93.22.27./index.html
An online Lesch–Nyhan group

Long Term Medical Conditions Alliance
Unit 212
16 Baldwins Gardens
London EC1N 7RJ
Tel: 020 7813 3637
Fax: 020 7813 3640
Website: www.lmca.org.uk
Campaigns to improve the quality of life of people with long-term medical conditions.

PUMPA – The Purine Metabolic Patients' Association
c/o Voluntary Services
Guy's Hospital
London Bridge
London SE1 9RT
Website: www.pumpa.co.uk
Information on all genetic metabolic disorders of purine and pyrimidine metabolism such as FJHN, LND and PRPS. Can put people in touch with each other, supports research and arranges annual seminars on different disorders in layman's language where patients play a key role. Proceedings are published and PUMPA collaborates with European experts from widely different disciplines to speed research.

REMAP
National Organiser
Hazeldene
Ightham, Sevenoaks
Kent TN15 9AD
Tel: 0845 1300 456
Fax: 0845 1300 789
Website: www.remap.org.uk
Makes or adapts aids, when not commercially available, for people with disabilities, at no charge to the disabled person. Local branches.

Society of Chiropodists and Podiatrists
1 Fellmongers' Path
Tower Bridge Road
London SE1 3LY
Tel: 020 7234 8620
Freephone: 0808 100 3883
Fax: 020 7234 8621
Website: www.feetforlife.org
Professional association. Provides a guide to foot problems and help in finding a local chiropodist.

General information and reference (UK)

British Dietetic Association
5th floor, Charles House
148–149 Great Charles Street
Birmingham B3 3HT
Tel: 0121 200 8080
Fax: 0121 200 8081
Website: www.bda.uk.com
Professional association supporting dietitians.

British Nutrition Foundation
High Holborn House
52–54 High Holborn
London WC1V 6RQ
Fax: 020 7404 6747
Website: www.nutrition.org.uk
Professional association. Does not offer information over the telephone; please send s.a.e.

British Society for Rheumatology
41 Eagle Street
London WC1R 4TL
Tel: 020 7242 3313
Fax: 020 7242 3277
Website:
www.rheumatology.org.uk
Administrative headquarters for various professional bodies. It does not have information for patients.

Genetic Interest Group
Unit 4d, Leroy House
436 Essex Road
London N1 3QP
Tel: 020 7704 3141
Fax: 020 7359 1447
Website: www.gig.org.uk
Umbrella organisation working with policy makers to benefit all people with genetic disorders by promoting awareness and encouraging discussion. Refers enquirers to support groups.

National Kidney Research Fund and Kidney Foundation
King's Chambers
Priesgate
Peterborough PE1 1FG
Tel: 01733 704650
Helpline: 0845 300 1499
Fax: 01733 704660
Website: www.nkrf.org.uk
Funds research into kidney transplantation techniques, patient welfare, renal units. Offers advice, information, support and grants, and refers to self-help groups.

Purine Research Unit
5th floor, Thomas Guy House
Guy's Hospital
London Bridge
London SE1 9RT
Tel: 020 7955 2438
Fax: 020 7955 4015
The first specialist laboratory in the UK, it tests and diagnoses cases of gout and inborn errors of metabolism; it also offers DNA tests.

Some reliable health websites

WebMD
www.my.webmd.com
A large US website from a company called Healthwise, Incorporated.

BBC Health
www.bbc.co.uk/health
Go to: 'ask_doctor' or 'Health and conditions' → 'arthritis' → 'links and organisations'.

Discovery Health Channel
www.health.discovery.com
Once in the website, click on 'Diseases and conditions, a to z' or just search for 'gout'.

Family Village
www.familyvillage.wisc.edu
Has 'message board' for families of recently diagnosed patients. Very useful for LNS and other purine metabolic disorders. Go to 'Library' from the homepage, look up in A to Z list.

Medhelp
www.medhelp.org/index.htm
US not-for-profit organisation, answers questions posed over the internet; sponsored by the Cleveland Clinic and Schering Oncology/Biotech.

The Times
www.thetimes.co.uk
Go to 'Medical Q&A' then 'A to Z'.

Websites of professional and learned societies and databases

Arthritis Foundation
www.arthritis.org
US site, providing much useful information on gout, diet and prescription drugs. Go to 'Conditions' → 'Disease Center' → 'G' to get information on gout and link to a brochure that can be read online or ordered by mail in the USA.

British Inherited Metabolic Disease Group (BIMDG)
www.bimdg.org.uk
For professionals such as dietitians, doctors, geneticists and others, as well as experts in metabolic disease.

European Academy of Childhood Disability
www.eacd-org.org
Professional association involving 35 European countries. Arranges meetings to encourage research and teaching in the healthcare professions. For doctors only.

European Society for the Study of Purine and Pyrimidine Metabolism in Man (ESSPPMM)
www.amg.gda.pl/~essppmm
A forum for doctors and researchers at every level, which includes information on metabolic disorders, and a list of diagnostic services available for purine and pyrimidine metabolic disorders and contacts in 19 EU countries.

National Institute of Arthritis and Musculoskeletal and Skin Diseases
www: niams.nih.gov
Professional US site, with information on gout topics.

Purine Research Society (USA)
www2.dgsys.com/~purine
US site, providing information on metabolic pathways, and a contact (www.gout-haters.com) to a pair of books with US-style recipes for low-purine food.

Society for the Study of Inborn Errors of Metabolism
www.ssiem.org.uk
Professional society with some useful links; for all involved in diagnosing and researching metabolic diseases.

*Suppliers of benzbromarone (Desuric) and of probenecid**

The following companies can supply drugs that are no longer manufactured in the UK. They require a doctor's prescription on a 'named patient' basis and an import licence. Advice is for professionals only; no information is provided for patients.

John Bell & Croyden
50–54 Wigmore Street
London W1U 2AU
Tel: 020 7935 5555
Fax: 020 7935 9605
Website:
www.johnbellcroyden.co.uk

IDIS World Medicines *
Millbank House
171–185 Ewell Road
Surbiton
Surrey KT6 6AX
Tel: 020 8410 0700
Fax: 020 8410 0800
Website: idispharma.co.uk

Welbeck Pharmaceuticals & Hospital Supplies*
39 Marylebone High Street
London W1U 4QG
Tel: 020 7935 4050
Fax: 020 7486 1054
Website: www.welbeckdrugs.com

Appendix 2
Useful Publications

Books for you

Caring for Children with Lesch–Nyhan Disease: a guide for parents and professionals, edited by Dr G McCarthy, published by PUMPA in conjunction with Chailey Heritage Clinical Services, London (2002) [Obtainable from PUMPA, contact details in Appendix 1.]

Gout: the patrician malady, by Roy Porter and George Rousseau, published by Yale University Press, New Haven CT (1998) [A historical survey of the disorder, its incidence, treatment, and society's attitude.]

The Patient's Internet Handbook, by Robert Kiley and Elizabeth Graham. Marston Books/Royal Society of Medicine Press, London (2001). [Available through bookstores or by phoning 01235 465500.]

Recipe books

Delia's How To Cook, Book 3, by Delia Smith, published by BBC Books, London (2001) [Chapter 5, 'Waist Watchers', has sensible advice and very attractive recipes that can be guaranteed to work.]

Dr Atkins Quick and Easy New Diet Cookbook, by RC Atkins and V Atkins, published by Pocket Books, London (2001) [Low-carbohydrate recipes and advice on weight loss; the regimen was controversial when low-fat diets were recommended but some elements of the Atkins diet are now widely accepted by nutritionists.]

Eat to Beat the Menopause, by Linda Kearns, published by Thorsons, London (1999) [Includes a recipe for the famous 'beat the menopause' cake, rich in nuts and seeds but no dairy products or added sugar.]

The Everyday Diabetic Cookbook, by Stella Bowling, published by Grub Street/Diabetes UK, London (2001) [Especially good for overweight people who are concerned about developing Type 2 diabetes.]

The Everyday Light-hearted Cookbook, by Anne Lindsay, published by Grub Street/British Heart Foundation, London (2001) [Gives principles for looking after the health of your heart but also applies generally.]

The Healthy Kitchen, by Dr Andrew Weil and Rosie Daley, published by Ebury Press, London (2002) [Has a wide range of recipes, with attractive illustrations.]

Natural Alternatives to HRT Cookbook, by Marilyn Grenville, published by Kyle Cathie, London (2000) [Many attractive recipes, low in meat and high in phyto-oestrogens, but be wary of dependence on soya products.]

Books for your doctor

Inherited Metabolic Diseases, by G Hoffmann, WL Nyhan, J Zschocke, SG Kahler and E Mayatepek, published by Lippincott Williams & Wilkins, Philadelphia PA (2002) [Signs, symptoms and differential diagnosis, with a solid clinical base.]

Physician's Guide to the Laboratory Diagnosis of Metabolic Diseases, 2nd edition, edited by N Blau, M Duran, ME Blaskovics and KM Gibson, published by Springer-Verlag, Berlin, Heidelberg, New York (2002) [Includes a comprehensive chapter on the purine metabolic disorders.]

Index

Note Page numbers in *italic* refer to diagrams or tables; numbers followed by '*g*' refer to entries in the Glossary.

Have you found **Gout – the 'at your fingertips' guide** practical and useful? If so, you may be interested in other books from Class Publishing.

High blood pressure – the 'at your fingertips' guide
SECOND EDITION £14.99
Dr Julian Tudor Hart, Dr Tom Fahey and Professor Wendy Savage
The authors use all their years of experience as blood pressure experts to answer over 340 real questions on high blood pressure, including questions you may feel uneasy about asking your doctor, as well as offering positive, practical advice on every aspect of your blood pressure.

Stop that heart attack!
SECOND EDITION £14.99
Dr Derrick Cutting
The easy, drug-free and medically accurate way to cut dramatically your risk of having a heart attack. Even if you already have heart disease, you can halt and even reverse its progress by following Dr Cutting's simple steps. Don't be a victim – take action NOW!

Diabetes – the 'at your fingertips' guide
FIFTH EDITION £14.99
Professor Peter Sonksen, Dr Charles Fox and Sue Judd
Over 460 questions on diabetes are answered clearly and accurately – the ideal reference book for everyone with diabetes.

Stroke – the 'at your fingertips' guide
£14.99
Dr Anthony Rudd, Penny Irwin and Bridget Penhale
This essential guidebook tells you all about strokes – and, most importantly, how to recover from them. As well as providing clear explanations of the medical processes, tests and treatments, the book is full of practical advice, including recuperation plans. You will find it inspiring.

Heart health – the 'at your fingertips' guide
SECOND EDITION £14.99
Dr Graham Jackson
This practical handbook, written by a leading cardiologist, answers all your questions about heart conditions. It tells you all about you and your heart; how to keep your heart healthy – or, if it has been affected by heart disease, how to make it as strong as possible.

Cancer – the 'at your fingertips' guide
THIRD EDITION £14.99
Val Speechley and Maxine Rosenfield
This invaluable reference guide gives you clear and practical information about cancer. Whether you have cancer yourself or are caring for someone who does, you will find in this book the information you need to reassure yourself, and enable you to take control.

Dementia: Alzheimer's and other dementias – the 'at your fingertips' guide
SECOND EDITION £14.99
Harry Cayton, Dr Nori Graham and Dr James Warner
At last – a book that tells you everything you need to know about Alzheimer's and other dementias. It is an invaluable contribution to understanding all forms of dementia.

Beating depression – the 'at your fingertips' guide £14.99
Dr Stefan Cembrowicz and Dr Dorcas Kingham
Depression is one of most common illnesses in the world – affecting up to one in four people at some time in their lives. Beating depression shows sufferers and their families that they are not alone, and offers tried and tested techniques for overcoming depression.